Gender-Specific Treatment

Gender-Specific Treatment

A Program for Chemically

Dependent Women in Recovery

Second Edition

Diane Dempsey Marr

Learning Publications, Inc.
Holmes Beach, Florida

ISBN 1-55691-230-7

© 1994, 2003 by Diane Dempsey Marr

All rights reserved. No part of this book may be reproduced or transmitted in any form or by any means, electronic or mechanical, including photocopying and recording, or by any information or retrieval systems, without permission in writing from the publisher.

Learning Publications, Inc.
5351 Gulf Drive
P.O. Box 1338
Holmes Beach, FL 34218-1338

Printing: 5 4 3 2 1   Year: 07 06 05 04 03

Illustrated by Dargan H. Marr

Printed in the United States of America.

Dedication

In each of our lives there are a few special people who manage to touch our hearts in a way no other could. In my life, one such person has been my cousin, Dina Marie. Throughout our childhood together she freely gave unconditional love and laughter. In adulthood, her demonstration of courage has earned my deepest respect. To her, and women like her, I dedicate this work.

Contents

Introduction ix
Session 1 1
Session 2 11
Session 3 23
Session 4 35
Session 5 43
Session 6 51
Session 7 59
Session 8 65
Appendix A–1 Problem Situation Handouts 73
Appendix A–2 Role Plays 75
Appendix A–3 Game Cards and Sorry Cards 79
Appendix A–4 Voting Cards 87
Appendix A–5 Handouts 89
Appendix B – Overheads 97
Appendix C – Illustration 101
Appendix D – Related Exercises 103
Appendix E – References 111

Acknowledgments

Although it is impossible to thank each person individually, I would like to voice my appreciation to all those who supported this project. I am truly grateful to the women in recovery who contributed through their willingness to be transparent and share a part of themselves. I would like to thank my colleagues, Drs. Stephanie Tovey, Thomas Fairchild, and M. Bryce Fifield for providing valuable comments with regard to the intervention's development and contents. A special thanks to director, Jeanne Iverson, and her wonderful staff at Whitman County Alcohol Center for their confidence and enthusiasm that kept me going despite occasional obstacles. I would like to extend a grateful heart to my husband, Dargan, who gave freely of himself throughout this endeavor in the form of technical assistance, artistic talent, and loving support. Finally, I would like to acknowledge my appreciation of the work of Thomas D'Zurilla and Marvin Goldfried (1971). Their conceptual model of skills training in problem solving influenced me in the development of the intervention program presented in this manual.

Introduction

We all face problems. They are a normal everyday part of life. Being prepared to deal with life's difficulties is important to us all. Despite this fact, many of us lack an organized and consistently effective way to approach our problems. Chemically dependent women are no exception. Instead of dealing with their problems, most turned to their drugs for relief. In recovery, chemically dependent women face an accumulation of problems that have built up during their addiction. They have come to admit that their pretreatment mode of coping failed to work for them. Now they need a new and more effective way to cope. It makes sense that taking a thoughtful and organized approach to problem solving would not only increase the chance for successful problem resolution, but would also strengthen their confidence in themselves and their ability to cope. That is what intervention in the lives of women with chemical problems should be all about.

The following summary of the intervention model offered here describes its organization of sessions in a way that is rational—an organization that fits with the experiences of many clinicians. Specifically designed for chemically dependent women in recovery, the problem-solving model you are about to teach is simple, straightforward, and easy to use in everyday living situations. The women you instruct will have the opportunity to learn an organized and informed approach to solving the problems they will face outside of treatment. The model is constructed to equip chemically dependent women with tools to face the challenges that lie ahead in their recovery.

Perhaps the greatest advantage of the model is its use of sample problem situations that are relevant to recovering women. These samples were generated through a survey of treatment providers and women in recovery. From the survey, major problem areas for chemically dependent women were identified and sample problems for each of these areas were formulated. Thus, sample situations used to teach problem-solving skills are particularly relevant to chemically dependent women in recovery.

The entire problem-solving model is presented over a span of eight sessions, with each session lasting 90 minutes. An outline of any individual session includes:

- the concept(s) to be taught,

- a session overview, and
- a list of materials needed to teach the session.

Detailed session format, directions, and instructional materials are provided for each of the eight sessions. A number of approaches and activities are used to maintain interest and promote learning.

Designed to teach the basic concepts of the problem-solving model, the approaches include lecture presentations, modeling, role play, visualization, group discussion, and group exercises. In addition, informal homework assignments are used to enhance between-session acquisition of skills and generalization of skills to real-life situations (Marr and Fairchild 1993).

Outline of the Model*

Step One: Familiarization
1. Acknowledgment and acceptance that problem situations are a common occurrence in daily living.
2. Recognition and identification of problem situations as they occur.
3. Restraint of automatic responses to problem situations.

Step Two: Systematic Definition
1. Dissect the problem into manageable concrete units, operationally defining each unit.
2. Through exploration of all aspects of the problem:
   a. Differentiate important from unimportant information.
   b. Establish appropriate goals.
   c. Explore subproblems and potential conflicts.
3. Gather additional information, if necessary.
4. Clearly state the problem.

Step Three: Production of Alternatives
1. Brainstorm a number of alternative solutions.

---
*Adapted from a model first developed by Thomas D'Zurilla and Marvin Goldfried (1971).

Step Four: Evaluation of Alternatives and Decision
1. Exploration of the potential outcomes of alternatives.
2. Gather additional information, if necessary.
3. Arrange alternative solutions in a hierarchy according to perceived effectiveness.
4. Choose an alternative.

Step Five: Confirmation of Choice
1. Gather information about actual outcome and consequences of the alternative chosen.
2. Make a critical evaluation of the consequences of the choice.
3. If goals have been met, exit the problem-solving model. If goals have not been met, return to an earlier appropriate step of problem-solving model.

Session Overview

Concept: Familiarization

- Acknowledgment and acceptance of problem situations as a common occurrence in daily living.
- Recognition and identification of problem situations as they occur.
- Restraint of automatic responses to problem situations.

Session Objectives

- The client will be able to recognize contributing factors in the daily living problems of the general population of women, as well as chemically dependent women in recovery.
- The client will be able to recognize nonproductive attitudes and beliefs that inhibit positive problem-solving behaviors.
- The client will recognize that problem situations are a normal part of daily living.
- The client will be able to cultivate a positive attitude toward self in terms of the ability to independently and successfully solve problems.

Session Format

1. Opening exercise
2. Introduction to the problem-solving model
    a. Rationale
    b. Description of model
    c. Expected benefits resulting from use of the model
3. Discussion of contributing factors in the daily living problems of chemically dependent women
4. Discussion of typical thoughts and reactions to problem situations
5. Problems as an expected occurrence
    a. Problems in daily living
    b. Problems in interpersonal relationships
    c. Chemically dependent women coping effectively and independently with problem situations

6. Closure of the session
   a. Summary
   b. Reminder of next scheduled meeting

Materials Needed

- Lecture notes
- Blackboard, chalk and eraser, or large sheets of paper, markers, and tacks

■ Opening Exercise (approximate time: 20 minutes)

Introduction Exercise: Introduce yourself to the group members. Ask each person to choose one other member to talk with briefly about: where the member is from, how they came to be in the group, and what they hope to accomplish in group. After the women are finished sharing, request that each person introduce to the group the member they just visited with.

Ground Rules: Briefly outline the following group parameters. These should be shared in a positive manner as the parameters are meant to facilitate group cooperation and cohesiveness.

- What goes on in group, stays in group.
- Attendance at each session is very important. Ask members to plan to attend all sessions.
- Support of others is welcome. Constructive criticism used to facilitate work is acceptable. Negativism and criticism of another member's work inhibits group growth and is discouraged.

★ At the end of the discussion concerning ground rules, give members a chance to ask questions.

■ Introduction to the Problem-Solving Model (approximate time: 10 minutes)

a. Rationale
b. Description of model
c. Expected benefits resulting from use of the model

Materials Needed

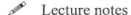 Lecture notes

Lecture Format: Below, a sample lecture is provided for you. Its content covers the major points outlined above. You may use the lecture verbatim or you can use your own words to convey the information. If you choose to use your own words, be careful to cover the major content and themes that are contained in the sample lecture.

Sample Lecture: *During the eight sessions we will spend together, we will be learning some specific problem-solving skills. This may sound rather funny since we all face problems on a daily basis. Certainly at our age we have had enough practice and know how to solve problems. But often times, the way we deal with a problem situation isn't always effective. For example, we might choose a solution quickly because it seemed like the thing to do at the time only to find out later that a bigger mess resulted from our choice . . . throwing the baby out with the bath water so to speak. Or we may have chosen to ignore the problem only to discover at a later date that the problem that was once the size of a small kitten is now looking more like a rather large, ill-tempered lion. Our best intentions to solve problem situations don't always work out the way we had hoped for.*

Chemically dependent women in recovery face numerous problems which demand solutions. We live in a world that is not only challenging in and of itself but also a world that is complicated by the results of our addictions. Often times, we may become so overwhelmed by the demands of daily living . . . family, job, financial responsibilities . . . that it appears there are no workable solutions to our dilemmas. The world seems to be working against us. We feel isolated and alone. We may lose our perspective. We may lose our confidence. We surely lose the healthy balance needed to achieve success in daily living. Somehow we must improve upon our management of daily living problems and either develop the confidence we never had or reclaim the confidence we lost. We know now that hiding behind our drugs is not the answer. What we once looked to as easy solutions to life's discomforts . . . our drugs . . . have turned out, instead, to be one of life's major problems. We need a new way to cope . . . and succeed.

The problem-solving model I am about to share with you will give you new tools to deal with problematic situations. The model can be applied to everyday living problems, including problems in your relationships with other people. The model is simple, straightforward, and easy to use. It has five steps.

Step 1. Recognize the problem

Lesson Plan

Step 2. Define the problem

Step 3. Generate solutions to the problem

Step 4. Choose a solution

Step 5. Evaluate your choice

Today we will take a general look at how problems develop and explore some problems common to all of us. In later sessions we will learn to recognize a problem when it occurs. We will also learn the in's and out's of defining problems, an important step in the model. A clear definition to any problem will help us to get a good grip on what we are dealing with. Without a definition how can we be sure what we need to solve? Next, we will learn some ways to generate as many solutions to a problem as possible. This third step can be fun and entertaining because this is the "anything goes" step. Bold, daring, and zany solutions are encouraged. In the fourth step we will learn to wade through and evaluate the solutions we came up with in Step 3, choosing the one we think will work best. And finally, we will learn how to evaluate the effectiveness of our choice. Did the solution do the job? If not, what else can be done?

Learning the problem-solving model will give you new tools for success. Rather than relying on old ways that didn't always work, you will have the opportunity to use these new skills in the challenges that lie ahead in your recovery. I believe that learning problem-solving skills will increase your ability to cope with problems in daily living and in your relationships with others.

Facing life without drugs can be scary because we used drugs to cope. We can look forward to challenges that help us grow beyond today by gaining confidence in our ability to handle whatever problems come our way . . . without the use of drugs.

■ Discussion of Contributing Factors in the Daily Living Problems of Chemically Dependent Women (approximate time: 10 minutes)

Materials Needed

🖉 Blackboard, chalk and eraser, or large sheets of paper, markers, and tacks

Large Group Discussion Format: Facilitate group exploration of factors that create or compound common problem situations in the lives of all women. Then help the group to focus in on factors that create or compound problem situations that are more specific to chemically dependent women. As ideas are shared, record them on the blackboard under the two separate categories: **All Women** and **Chemically Dependent Women.**

Make sure to reinforce members' attempts to share. Model appropriate group participation by offering several ideas yourself. Below are some examples of possible factors.

All Women	Chemically Dependent Women
• Changing roles of women	• Husband who drinks heavily
• Childcare	• Little family support for recovery
• Health issues	• Old friends want you to go drinking with them
• Dealing with a difficult boss	

■ Discussion of Typical Thoughts and Reactions to Problem Situations (approximate time: 15 minutes)

Materials Needed

🖉 Blackboard, chalk and eraser, or large sheets of paper, markers, and tacks

Large Group Discussion Format: Lead the group in an informal sharing time in which members have the opportunity to explore how they may be reacting to problem situations in self-defeating ways, both cognitively and emotionally. Lead questions brought before the group should focus on the following:

- What do you tell yourself when a problem does occur?
- What do you choose to do when you are faced with a problem?
- What part of your attempts to solve the problem work for you?
- Which of your beliefs or actions don't work well for you? Why don't they work well for you?

Share one way you have dealt with problems that did not work well for you. Frame the example in the formatted questions above.

Below are some examples of self-defeating approaches to problem solving.

- I don't do anything and hope the problem will go away.
- I try to forget about the problem. After a few drinks the problem doesn't seem so big anymore.
- I chalk it up to bad luck.
- I think its not fair and feel sorry for myself.
- I do the first thing that pops into my head and hope the problem will get better.
- I am overwhelmed by problems. If I was a better person, these problems wouldn't come into my life.
- I get mad at my family. If they would only do what I want them to do, I wouldn't have these problems.

■ Problems as an Expected Occurrence (approximate time: 30 minutes)

a. Problems in daily living

b. Problems in interpersonal relationships

c. Chemically dependent women coping effectively and independently with problem situations

Materials Needed

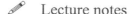 Lecture notes

Lecture Format: Below, a sample lecture is provided for you. Its' content covers the major points outlined above. You may use the lecture verbatim or you may use your own words to convey the information. If you choose to use your own words, be careful to cover the major content and themes that are contained in the sample lecture.

Group Exercise: Following the lecture presentation, members will practice seeing themselves as effective and independent problem solvers. A visualization exercise is provided for this purpose. Be sure to **slowly read this exercise verbatim, using a calm reassuring tone.** Pacing is a very important aspect of relaxation and visualization. The entire visualization exercise should take approximately 10 to 15 minutes.

Sample Lecture: *Maybe you prefer the ostrich approach and try to hide from your problems. But did you ever notice that when you pulled*

your head out of its hiding place, your problem was still there waiting for you? Or maybe you would like to believe that your problems will go away when your bad luck does. Are you still wondering when your luck is going to change? The fact of the matter is that problems are a normal and expected part of everyday living. That's right . . . normal and expected. As sure as the sun comes up you can bet that something or someone out there is waiting to challenge your patience and your creative problem-solving abilities. It may be the washing machine, your boss, a bounced check written by your beloved spouse, a pleasant note from the IRS reminding you that your taxes are late, or a car with no gas.

Regardless of how your problems present themselves, there is no doubt that they will continue to appear. Furthermore, problems come to visit each and every one of us. There is no one person who remains problem free if they are alive and breathing. If you ever believed you had met someone who was problem free, chances are that they were either dead, heavily into denial, or . . . an expert and enthusiastic problem solver.

Just because we quit using drugs does not mean that we will be problem free. As chemically dependent women, we face many problem situations. Some of these problem situations are a part of normal everyday living (sometimes made worse as a result of our addiction). Other problems are a direct result of our drug use. Coping effectively and independently with problem situations is possible, not just for the woman next door but for the rest of us as well. We have the ability to face each problem as it comes and find workable solutions. In recovery, we have hope for a better future and begin to believe in our ability to succeed, drug free. We will face the challenge of finding new solutions to old problems. Using a well thought-out strategy to find those solutions is an important step towards success.

Visualization Exercise

Directions: I would like to invite everybody to participate in a little experiment with me. We are going to try something that will help you learn to see yourselves as effective problem solvers. It is called visualization. All you have to do is follow my directions. Are you ready? First, I want you to make yourselves as comfortable as possible. Find a relaxed position. Take your shoes off if that helps. . . . Good. Now close your eyes, here we go.

Exercise: *Keeping your eyes closed, I want you to take a few deep breaths . . . slowly breathe in . . . and . . . breathe out . . . inhale . . . exhale. Good. Breathe in . . . and . . . breathe out . . . inhale . . . exhale. That's* *right. With each breath you feel yourself becoming more and more relaxed . . . more and more calm. . . . Inhale. . . . Exhale. Good. . . . Nothing can disturb your sense of peace . . . and tranquility . . . Nothing can bother you. . . . There are no pressing matters. . . . Nothing that needs your attention. . . . You are free to relax . . . and enjoy the calm peacefulness. . . . With each passing moment . . . you find yourself . . . more . . . and more . . . relaxed. . . . Tension is leaving your body . . . slowly draining away . . . with each breath you feel more . . . and more comfortable . . . more calm. . . . Time loses all meaning for you. . . . It no longer matters . . . as you feel the peacefulness gently come over you. . . . You are now entering a different world. . . . The road is easy to travel . . . because you feel . . . calm . . . relaxed . . . and successful in the new world. . . . Let your mind take you there. . . . This is your special place where you feel . . . peace and serenity surround you . . . hugging your body . . . your very being. Take a look around you and notice the sights . . . the smells . . . and the sounds. . . . What a wonderful place this is . . . so quiet . . . and so peaceful. Enjoy the relaxing atmosphere of your special place. . . . In your special place . . . you can deal with anything that happens. . . . Relaxed. . . . Confident. . . . Calm. . . . Experience the good feelings of success and mastery. . . . Nothing is impossible. . . . You can take care of whatever comes your way. . . . When you see a problem coming. . . . You are . . . very calm . . . calm and peaceful. . . . Confident that you can take care of the problem. . . . Look. Here comes a problem now . . . and it is demanding your attention. . . . It is a big . . . sticky problem . . . but you are not worried. . . . You can handle it. . . . And you do . . . it feels good to take care of things and move on . . . skilled . . . confident . . . sure of yourself. You did so well. . . . You can feel good about your abilities . . . relaxed . . . successful. . . . Now its time to leave your special place. . . . Remember . . . you can come back whenever you want . . . You can bring back the good feelings you had in your special place. . . . Peacefulness. . . . Strength. . . . Confidence. . . . Success. . . . Slowly come back . . . as you become more and more aware of your breathing . . . inhale . . . exhale . . . breathe in . . . breathe out. . . . Once again . . . it is time to come back. At the count of five . . . I want you to open your eyes . . . one . . . two . . . three . . . four . . . five. . . . Now open your eyes.*

Directions: Give the group members a few moments to re-orient themselves. Invite members to comment on their experience. Use the following comments to put closure on the exercise:

You can use this kind of exercise whenever you have a problem that demands your attention. All it takes is a few quiet moments of privacy. Us-

ing visualization helps you to relax and see yourself coping with problems in a positive way. It can help to increase your confidence and chances for success. Between now and our next session, you may want to practice your own visualization exercise.

■ Closure of the Session (approximate time: 5 minutes)

    a.   Summary

    b.   Reminder of next scheduled meeting

Summary: Briefly summarize the major points covered in the body of Session 1 (#2 through #4). Ask members if they have any questions.

★ The facilitator may way want to make tapes of the visualization exercise and send a tape home with each member.

Session Overview

Concept: Familiarization
- Acknowledgment and acceptance that problem situations are a common occurrence in daily living.
- Recognition and identification of problem situations as they occur.
- Restraint of automatic responses to problem situations.

Session Objectives
- The client will be able to identify the general problem area of a problem situation.
- The client will be able to identify the underlying concerns of a problem situation.
- The client will be able to identify who owns the problem.
- The client will be able to inhibit automatic responses to the problem situation.

Session Format
1. Introduction
   a. Review of Session 1
   b. Overview of Session 2
2. Identification of general areas in which problems can occur for chemically dependent women.
   a. List areas
   b. Underlying concerns that create problem situations
3. Recognition of the Problem
   a. Identification
   b. Inhibition of automatic responses
4. Review of major points in Step 1 of the problem-solving model
   a. Problems as a normal occurrence
   b. Chemically dependent women in recovery dealing effectively with problems
   c. Identifying the problem
   d. Restraint of automatic responses

5. Integration of knowledge
    a. Practicing the four major points in Step 1 of the problem-solving model
6. Closure of the session
    a. Summary
    b. Homework assignment

Materials Needed

- Lecture notes
- Blackboard, chalk and eraser, or large sheets of paper, markers, and tacks
- Handouts
- Pencils
- Overhead #1 (Appendix C)

- **Introduction (approximate time: 10 minutes)**
    a. Review of Session 1
    b. Overview of Session 2

Review: Summarize the major points covered in Session 1. You can use the overview of the session below for this purpose.

Session 1 Review

1. Discussion of contributing factors in the daily living problems of chemically dependent women
2. Discussion of typical thoughts and reactions to problem situations
3. Problems as an expected occurrence
    a. Problems in daily living
    b. Problems in interpersonal relationships
    c. Chemically dependent women coping effectively and independently with problem situations

Ask group members if they have any questions or comments. Solicit any input they may have concerning the practice they may have engaged in outside of group time with the visualization exercise.

Overview: Review the major points that will be covered in Session 2. You can use the overview of the session for this purpose. Step 1 of the problem-solving model will be completed at the end of this session.

- **Identification of General Areas in Which Problems Can Occur for Chemically Dependent Women (approximate time: 15 minutes)**
    a. General areas
    b. Underlying concerns that create problem situations.

Materials Needed

- Blackboard, chalk and eraser, or large sheets of paper, markers, and tacks
- Problem situation handouts (Appendix A-1)

Group Discussion and Problem Situation Handouts: Lead the group in a brief discussion of the points outlined above. Make two separate

Lesson Plan

lists for points 'a' and 'b.' on the blackboard, recording group input. Below is a sample list for both points.

General Problem Areas	Underlying Concerns
• Recovery • Finances • Employment • Parenting • Marriage • Family	• Competing goals • Competing demands • Differing needs • Change in the usual • Trying out new behavior affects relationships with others

After you have completed a brief list, read each of the two problem situation handouts provided. For each situation, have the group identify the problem and the underlying concerns(s) that may have created the problem. Allow for different opinions to enhance the discussion. This will assist group members in exploring alternative frames of reference.

📄 Use problem situation handouts in Appendix A-1 here.

■ Recognition of the Problem
Approximate time: 20 minutes

    a.   Identification

    b.   Inhibition of automatic responses

Materials Needed

- Lecture notes
- Role-play cards (Appendix A-2)

Lecture and Roleplay Format: A brief lecture presentation covering the major points outlined above will be followed by role-play situations. Again, a sample lecture has been provided for you below. Its content covers the major points outlined above. You may use the lecture verbatim or you can use your own words to convey the information. If you choose to use your own words, be careful to cover the major content and themes that are contained in the sample lecture. Role-play cards are also provided. Ask for a volunteer from the group to help you with each of the situations. After each role play, explore the questions written on the roleplay card with group members.

Sample Lecture: *We have just explored some of the general areas in which problems can occur and possible concerns that may be behind those problems. Now we are going to take a look at how we can improve our ability to identify problems more accurately. We will work on solving them later. For now, we just want to identify them. Some problems are more easily identified than others. For example, its easy to figure out that we have a problem if we come home to find our dog treading water in a flooded laundry room or if we run out of gas on an isolated road at night. Not all problems are so obvious though. Before its too late, how can we identify those problems that always seem to sneak up on us? Or what about the problem that seems to never end despite our best efforts? How can we identify the real issue so we can find a solution that finally works? There are ways to deal with both of these types of problems.*

Let's look at the sneaky problem first. Perhaps that problem isn't so sneaky after all. Remember the ostrich? It could be that we chose to ignore or hide from this problem when it first showed up.

Solution: *When we find ourselves wanting to play the ostrich, we need to stop and take the time to identify the problem. We also need to make mental notes of the obvious warning signs of an up-and-coming problem situation. If we are alert and stand our ground problems will take us by surprise less often.*

*Now let's explore the other situation. The problem that never goes away can be very discouraging and, worse yet, wear on our patience too. Perhaps we have decided that the problem belongs to us and it does not belong to us. When attempting to identify a problem situation we should **always** ask ourselves: Who owns this problem? If it does not belong to us then we are not the ones who have control over the solution. For example, our father's drinking is a problem. But do we own the problem? No. Our father does. We cannot make him stop drinking. Remember that only the person who owns the problem can fix the problem.*

The other possibility for the never-ending problem is that we never took the time to properly explore solutions. Instead, we made a series of quick choices that never solved the problem. We forgot to stop and think things through.

Our feelings and thoughts are great problem barometers. Paying better attention to them can help us to identify problems. Being aware of thoughts and feeling can also help us to stop and think instead of making a quick decision about the solution to the problem. Taking the time to better know ourselves in this area is worth the effort. What are some thoughts and feelings that tell us a problem is about to happen or has already happened?

If you are unsure of the answer to this question, I would like to encourage you to begin finding the answer. We will take a look at some sample situations that other chemically dependent women have found to be problems in their lives. Pay special attention to what you are thinking and feelings as the situation is described. Then try your hand at identifying the problems in each situation. Remember, you are not looking for solutions right now. You don't want to jump to any conclusions.

📄 Use role-play cards in Appendix A-2 here.

■ Review of the Major Points in Step 1 of the Problem-Solving Model (approximate time: 5 minutes)

   a. Problems as a normal occurrence
   b. Chemically dependent women in recovery dealing effectively with problems
   c. Identifying the problem
   d. Restraint of automatic responses

Materials Needed

   ✎ Lecture notes

Lecture Format: The purpose of this presentation is to give the women a clear and concise overview of Step 1 which deals with the concept of familiarization. Below, a sample lecture has been provided for you. Its content covers the major points outlined above. You may use the lecture verbatim or you can use your own words to convey the information. If you choose to use your own words, be careful to cover the major content and themes that are contained in the sample lecture.

Sample Lecture: *As recovering women, we will want to develop new approaches to coping with life's problems. Let's put together everything we've learned so far. Looking at the entire picture will help us to fine tune our skills.*

So far we have faced the fact that problems do happen. They happen to all of us. No one is exempt from problems, not even that nice lady that lives next to us. The occurrence of problems in our lives has nothing to do with fate or bad luck, but has everything to do with the fact that they are a normal part of life. At times, our problems seemed larger than life. Often, we made the problems worse with our drug use. Problems were a great excuse to drink.

I believe that each of us here today has learned that drinking and drugs are not the answers to difficulties we face. Fortunately, we can learn new and better ways to cope. Chemically dependent women in recovery can successfully solve problems—without drugs.

We've talked about and practiced how to identify a problem. When identifying problems remember to: 1) Pay attention to your feelings and thoughts. They are good problem barometers. Always make sure to take the time to explore thoughts and feelings. Try to determine what they are telling you. 2) Always ask yourself, "who owns the problem?" This can be confusing at times especially when you are upset. Take a few moments to calmly analyze the situation and circumstances. If you don't own the problem, then you need not try to fix it. 3) Finally, stop and think. Do not act on your first impulse. There is some groundwork to lay before you can choose the best solution for yourself. We'll talk more about that later.

■ Integration of Knowledge Approximate time: 35 minutes

    a.   Practicing the four major points in Step 1 of the problem-solving model

Materials Needed

- Overhead #1 (Appendix C)
- Handout #1 (Appendix B-5)
- Pencils

Modeling and Group Practice: After explaining the exercise and before giving them the handouts, use the model problem situation below to teach the behavior you want the members to use. Use Overhead #1 as a visual aid during the modeling exercise. After reading the situation aloud, verbalize the thought process you are engaging in to answer the questions at the bottom of the sample. Some possible answers are provided for you.

Working with a partner, group members will have the opportunity to identify several aspects of a problem situation. Use Session 2, Handout #1 (Appendix B-5), for this purpose. A copy of the problem situation on this handout is provided for you below. Included on your copy (but not on group members' copies) are some possible answers to the questions posed. Give the women approximately five minutes to work and then discuss the problem situation as a group. Record their answers on the blackboard.

Directions: I want you to pick a partner to work on a problem situation I will give you. Together, I want you to write down the following: a) what the main problem is, b) what the underlying concern(s) might be, and c) who owns the problem. Before we do this, I will demonstrate an example for you.

Model Problem Situation: Sandy has worked at her job for five years now. It has been a good experience and she has received a lot of positive attention for her efforts. Recently she has felt a little bored and wishes she could try something new. When her boss offers her a new and more challenging position in the company, Sandy has mixed feelings. Part of her is excited and happy. Another part of her is afraid. She is worried that she does not have the ability to do what her boss is asking. Sandy drives home after work consumed and upset by her mixed feelings. Although she has not drank in months, Sandy decides to have a glass of wine to calm her nerves. One drink leads to another and before she knows it, Sandy has finished the bottle of wine. The next morning Sandy returns to work and turns down the offer of a new position.

Question: What is the main problem?

Answer: Sandy wants a new position but did not take it. It doesn't appear that Sandy believes in her own abilities that were obvious to her boss. Low self-esteem.

Question: What are the underlying concerns?

Answer: Sandy has difficulty managing her feelings. She did not stop and think. By drinking, Sandy robbed herself of the opportunity to work through her feelings and understand them. Had she chosen the latter, she would have been in a better position to make a good decision for herself.

Question: Who owns the problem?

Answer: Sandy does!

📄 Give Handout #1 in Appendix B-5 to group members and read it aloud.

Below are the questions and some possible answers for Handout #1.

Problem Situation: Pat is an attractive brunette in her early forties. Since her divorce two years ago, she insists that variety is the all important ingredient in her social life, particularly in dating. Although Pat talks a good line, she is starting to wonder if her version of "variety" is all that great. She has lost count of the number of men she has dated and questions her decision to be intimate with most of them for brief periods of time. When she is honest with herself, she admits that most of the time she feels lonely and abandoned even when she is with one of her men. Pat attempts to erase her feelings of emptiness and fear with more men but the feelings never seem to stay away for long.

Question: What is the main problem?

*Answer: Pat is unhappy with her current choices around relationships. She has failed to **stop** and **think**. She continues to make the same choices that bring her unhappiness.*

Question: What are the underlying concerns?

Answer: Inability to establish or maintain intimate relationships. Fear of abandonment. Dependency.

Question: Who owns the problem?

Answer: Pat does.

★ If time permits, use the exercise below.

Visualization Exercise

Repeat the same exercise you facilitated in Session 1. Give the women some time to get comfortable and relaxed before starting the exercise. The entire exercise should take approximately 10 minutes. Below, directions are provided for you.

Directions: Since problems will continue to appear in our lives, we will practice a positive approach to problem solving. Today, I want to invite everybody to participate in the same visualization exercise we did during our last session. Remember that the exercise is designed to help you see yourselves as effective problem solvers. The more you practice, the better you will get at it, and the more effective it will be for you.

Again, all you have to do is follow my directions. Are you ready? First, I want you to get as comfortable as possible. Find the best position for you in the chair. You can take your shoes off if you like. . . . Good. Now close your eyes, here we go.

Exercise: *Keeping your eyes closed, I want you to take a few deep breaths . . . slowly breathe in . . . and . . . breathe out . . . inhale . . . exhale. Good. With each breath you feel yourself becoming more and more relaxed . . . more and more calm . . . inhale . . . exhale. . . . That's right . . . Nothing can disturb your sense of peace and . . . tranquility . . . nothing can bother you . . . there are no pressing matters . . . nothing that needs your . . . attention . . . you are free to relax and enjoy the calm . . . peacefulness. . . . With each passing moment . . . you . . . find yourself . . . more and more . . . relaxed. . . . Tension is leaving your body . . . slowly draining . . . away . . . with each breath you feel more and more . . . comfortable . . . more calm. Time loses all meaning for you . . . it no longer matters . . . as you feel the . . . peacefulness gently come over you. You are now entering a different world . . . the road is easy to travel . . . because you feel . . . calm . . . relaxed . . . and successful in the new world. Let your mind take you there . . . your special place where you feel peace and serenity surround you . . . hugging your body . . . your very being. Take a look around* *you and notice . . . the sights . . . the smells . . . and the sounds. What a wonderful place this is . . . so quiet and peaceful. Enjoy the relaxing atmosphere of your special place . . . in your special place you can deal with anything that happens . . . relaxed . . . confident . . . calm . . . experience the good feelings of success . . . and mastery . . . nothing is impossible . . . you can take care of whatever comes your way . . . when you see a problem coming . . . you are . . . calm and peaceful . . . confident that you can take care of the problem. And you do . . . it feels good to take care of things and move on . . . skilled . . . confident . . . sure of yourself. You did so well . . . you can feel good about your abilities . . . relaxed . . . successful. . . . And now its time to leave your special place . . . you can come back whenever you want . . . you can bring back the good feelings you had in your special place . . . peacefulness . . . strength . . . confidence . . . success. Slowly come back . . . as you become more and more aware of your breathing . . . once again . . . come back. At the count of five . . . I want you to open your eyes . . . one . . . two . . . three . . . four . . . five . . . now open your eyes.*

Directions: Give the group members a few moments to re-orient themselves. Invite any of the members who would like to comment on their experience to share with the group. Was their experience any different this time when compared to their first experience?

■ Closure of the Session (approximate time: 5 minutes)

    a.   Summary

    b.   Homework assignment

Summary: Briefly summarize the major points covered in the body of Session 2 (#2 through #6). Ask members if they have any questions.

Homework Assignment: Ask the group members to keep an informal journal. Before the next meeting, members should record several problem situations as they occur. Ask that they pay special attention to how they identified each situation as a problem. In particular, have them record feelings and thoughts that they experienced when each problem arose.

★ Remind members of the time and day of the next meeting.

Session Overview

Concept: Systematic Definition

- Dissect the problem into manageable concrete units, operationally defining each unit.
- Through exploration of all aspects of the problem:
  a. differentiate important from unimportant information,
  b. establish appropriate goals, and
  c. explore subproblems and potential conflicts.
- Gather additional information, if necessary.
- Clearly state the problem.

Session Objectives

- The client will be able to distinguish important from unimportant information.
- The client will be able to distinguish internal from external information and use each in defining the problem situation.
- The client will be able to identify aspects of the problem for which background information would prove helpful.
- The client will learn to use clear terminology, operationally defining terms used in describing the problem situation.

Session Format

1. Introduction
   a. Review of Session 2
   b. Overview of Session 3
2. Transitioning from problem identification to problem definition
   a. Differences between identification and definition
   b. How the two components work together
3. Making problems more manageable: breaking them down into concrete parts
   a. Identifying relevant information: external and internal events
   b. Exploring background information
4. Learning to clarify problems

a. Operationally defining terms
   b. Recognizing an impasse: when to seek more information
5. Closure of the session
   a. Summary
   b. Homework assignment

Materials Needed

- Lecture notes
- Blackboard, chalk and eraser, or large sheets of paper, markers, and tacks
- Handouts #2 and #3 (Appendix B-5)
- Overhead #1 (Appendix C)
- Pencils

■ Introduction (approximate time: 10 minutes)

Review: Summarize the major points covered in Session 2. You can use the overview of the session below for this purpose.

Session 2 Review

1. Identification of general areas in which problems can occur for chemically dependent women.
    a. List areas
    b. Underlying concerns that create problem situations
2. Recognition of the problem
    a. Identification
    b. Inhibition of automatic responses
3. Review of major points in Step 1 of the problem-solving model
    a. Problems as a normal occurrence
    b. Chemically dependent women in recovery dealing effectively with problems
    c. Identifying the problem
    d. Restraint of automatic responses
4. Integration of knowledge
    a. Practicing the four major points in Step 1 of the problem-solving model

Ask group members if they have any questions or comments. Solicit any input they may have about the homework assignment. How did the journal work for them?

Overview: Review the major points that will be covered in Session 3. You can use the overview of the session for this purpose. Learning Step 2 of the problem-solving model will begin with this lesson.

■ Transitioning from Problem Identification to Problem Definition (approximate time: 5 minutes)

    a. Differences between *identification* and *definition*
    b. How the two components work together

Lesson Plan

Materials Needed

✏ Lecture notes

Lecture Format: A brief lecture presentation covering the major points above will be used in the transition from Step 1 to Step 2 of the problem-solving model. A sample lecture has been provided for you below. Its content covers the major points outlined above. You may use the lecture verbatim or you can use your own words to convey the information. If you choose to use your own words, be careful to cover the major content and themes that are contained in the sample lecture.

Sample Lecture: *In our first two sessions we dealt with the first step in the problem-solving model, learning to identify a problem. Now we will begin the second step of the model: learning to define the problem we have identified. The difference between identifying and defining a problem is really a matter of degree. Identifying a problem is recognizing the existence of the problem. In saying that a problem does indeed exist, we can pinpoint what kind of problem it is and perhaps identify some of its underlying issues.*

When we want to define the problem, we go a step beyond identifying it and become more specific. We have looked at the problem in a general sort of way and now we want to break the problem into small parts so we can understand it better. Problem identification and definition fit together to give us a clearer picture of the specific problem situation we are dealing with. It is only with a clear picture that we can begin to search for solutions. Taking the necessary time to define our problems will increase our chance of finding a solution that we can be happy with. Today we will begin to work on developing skills to define problems.

■ Making Problems More Manageable: Breaking them Down into Concrete Parts (approximate time: 40 minutes)

a. Identifying relevant information: external and internal events

b. Exploring background information

Materials Needed

✏ Lecture notes

✏ Blackboard, chalk and eraser, or large sheets of paper, markers, and tacks

✎ Handout #2 (Appendix B-5)

✎ Overhead #1 (Appendix C)

Lecture, Modeling, and Group Exercise Format: You will now be teaching group members to break down problems into manageable parts by working through a sample problem situation. First, you will be giving the group some brief instructions on how to begin the process of problem definition. A sample lecture has been provided for you below. Its content covers the major points outlined above. You may use the lecture verbatim or you can use your own words to convey the information. If you choose to use your own words, be careful to cover the major content and themes that are contained in the sample lecture. After giving instructions, you will then model the desired behavior using the example that has been provided. Use Overhead #1 (Appendix C) as a visual aid. Finally, after passing out Handout #2 (Appendix B-5), group members will be given the opportunity to work through a problem situation.

Sample Lecture: *We know how to identify a problem situation. Now we will take a look at how we can define it. The first step in this process is to break down the problem into manageable parts. We can do this by identifying and separating out important from unimportant information. Important information is that information which is central to your problem.*

For example: Your child comes to you crying and says that she and her friend were playing house upstairs and having fun when the door slammed on her friend's finger and it is now bleeding. Unimportant information is that the children were playing house. Important information is that the friend is injured.

Important information comes to us in two forms: through external (or outside) events and internal (or inside) events. In our example, the external event would have been the report of an accident. Internal events might have been your thought that the child was in need of medical attention as well as your feelings of concern. External events are outward things we can identify while internal events are our thoughts and feelings.

After separating important from unimportant information, you should then gather background information on the important aspects of the problem. You want to have as much information as possible if you are going to get a clear definition of the problem.

Using our example of the two children again, you may want to ask the following questions to gather background information: What room were the children playing in? Which door slammed on the friend's finger? Was it a metal bi-fold door? A heavy sliding glass door? These questions would help you to locate the child and get a better idea of how bad the in-

jury might be. Background information gives us a framework to better understand the problem situation.

Do you remember the problem situation we used in our last session about Sandy? We left poor Sandy hanging. I am going to read her situation to you one more time and demonstrate what I have just been talking to you about. First I will try to separate important from unimportant information. Then I will identify some areas in which background information would help us to get a better picture of Sandy's problem. After I am finished demonstrating these two skills, I will give you a problem situation that we can work on as a group.

Directions: Using Overhead #1 (Appendix C), read the example aloud to the group. Then use the list below to identify for the group relevant and irrelevant information. Finally, using the list, provide the group with some areas in which background information would be useful.

Modeling Example: Sandy has worked at her job for five years now. It has been a good experience and she has received a lot of positive attention for her efforts. Recently she has felt a little bored and wishes she could try something new. When her boss offers her a new and more challenging position in the company, Sandy has mixed feelings. Part of her is excited and happy. Another part of her is afraid. She worries that she does not have the ability to do what her boss is asking. Sandy drives home after work consumed and upset by her mixed feelings. Although she has not drank in months, Sandy decides to have a glass of wine to calm her nerves. One drink leads to another and before she knows it, Sandy has finished the bottle of wine. The next morning Sandy returns to work and turns down the offer of a new position.

We have already identified the problem for Sandy. She wants a change but turned down the job offered to her. We thought that maybe poor self-esteem was an underlying concern.

Important Information

External:
— Sandy has done well in her present position.
— She wants a new position.
— She was offered a new position.
— After being abstinent, Sandy drank.
— She turned down the new position.

Internal:
- Sandy was feeling bored with her job.
- She had mixed feelings about the offer of a new position.
- Sandy was afraid she was not capable of doing the new job.

Unimportant Information

External:
- Sandy worked at her job for five years.
- The kind of wine Sandy drank.
- What Sandy wore that day.

Background Information:
- What has been going on with Sandy prior to the new job offer?
- What did the new position entail and would the company have provided training for Sandy?
- Does she have a clear picture of her true abilities?
- Sandy needed to deal with her mixed emotions in a better way. What are some other ways she has used in the past that would have proven more effective? Why didn't she use them in this situation?

Directions: Give group members Handout #2 (Appendix B-5). Read the example aloud to the group and then invite members to begin defining the problem. What appears to be important information (external and internal)? What appears to be unimportant information? Record members' responses on the blackboard.

A list of relevant and irrelevant information is provided for you. If they are missed, help group members to identify these examples in the problem situation. Welcome active discussion and involvement in the exercise. After the group has identified important components of the problem, ask them to generate a list of areas for which background information would be helpful. Again, a list is provided for you. If the areas contained in the list are missed, help group members to identify these examples in the problem situation.

Review of Handout #2 (Appendix A-5): Version One of Donna's Story

Donna has been staying home a lot lately. Since she quit using, Donna's daily routine includes: taking her two preschoolers to the babysitter's house in the green Ford she drives, going to work at the department store, picking the children up, running errands, returning home to cook for herself and her children, and staying home the remainder of the evening doing household chores. The exception to this routine occurs on Tuesday and Friday nights when Donna attends her 12-step group meetings. Usually she chooses to go straight home rather than go out for coffee with other members after the meetings. When Donna's old friends or family calls, she keeps conversations short and makes excuses for not visiting with them.

Donna feels tired, lonely, and scared. She worries that she will use again if she does not stay away from her old habits and old friends. Using again could mean that she would lose custody of her two young children. She could not bear this. People in her 12-step group have offered support but Donna's fear has walled her off from their help. Besides, Donna is uncomfortable with the people in her group. Even though attending has helped her to stay drug free, Donna doesn't want to get too involved. She thinks that a lot of the members are very religious and expect her to believe in God.

Important Information

External:

— All of Donna's time is spent in structured situations: home, work, and meetings.

— Donna spends minimum time socializing.

— Much of Donna's time is spent working.

— Donna does not have any play time away from responsibilities.

— Donna is avoiding people for various reasons.

— Donna's primary interactions are with her two children.

Internal:

— Donna is tired, scared, and lonely.

— She is afraid of losing her children.

Session 3   31

— Religion and God are subjects that Donna is uncomfortable with.

Unimportant information

External:

— What nights Donna attends meetings.

— What kind of job Donna has.

— What kind of car Donna drives.

Background Information:

— Why is Donna afraid of losing custody of her children?

— Why does she avoid old friends and family?

— Does she have a support system? If not, does she know how to create one?

— Does she have any leisure activities she used to enjoy or have any she would like to try?

■ Learning to Clarify Problems (approximate time: 30 minutes)

    a. Operationally defining terms

    b. Recognizing an impasse: when to seek more information

Materials Needed

- Lecture notes
- Blackboard, chalk and eraser, or large sheets of paper, markers, and tacks
- Handout #3 (Appendix B-5)
- Pencils

Lecture and Group Exercise Format: You will now give a brief presentation and then lead the group in an exercise that teaches members the difference between operational definitions and definitions that are unclear. A sample lecture has been provided for you below. You may use the lecture verbatim or you can use your own words to convey the information. If you choose to use your own words, be careful to cover the major content and themes that are contained in the sample lecture. After the presentation, pass out Handout #3 (Appendix B-5) to the group members.

They will use this handout along with Handout #2 (Appendix B-5) to practice operationally defining terms and problem situations.

After they complete the task, conduct a discussion on the results of their efforts. At the end of the discussion, make sure to emphasize the importance of clear definitions and how clarity enhances the problem-solving process.

Sample Lecture: *So far, we have been working with problems that have been clearly defined. Examples have supplied us with enough information to give us a good picture of the general overall situation. Now we are going to take a look at what happens when things are not so clear and information is missing. We will learn: a) the difference between clear definitions and vague or fuzzy descriptions of words, b) when to seek more information to help define a problem in a clear manner. Here is an example that is difficult to understand because of the terms used.*

Fuzzy: *Sue says that when Bob comes over to visit, he grosses her out. She would like to visit with him if he weren't so yucky.*

Its difficult to tell what is going on in this example. We need more information from Sue to understand the meaning of several terms.

Clear Definitions: *a) "grosses me out" translates to "I am uncomfortable and I don't want to be around him" and b) "yucky" translates to "Bob wears dirty clothes and smells like he has not bathed in some time."*

As you can see, defining the terms we use is very important if we, as well as others, expect to clearly understand the problem. Not only should terms be clear, but problems should also be defined in a way that makes it easy to understand the real problem. Listen to this example.

Fuzzy: *Marge wants to leave because her in-laws make her crazy.*

Clear Definition of the Problem Situation: *When Marge visits her in-laws, they make numerous comments about their son's appearance: how wrinkled his clothes look, how thin and tired he appears, and how unhappy he seems since she has returned to work. Marge believes they are putting pressure on her to fill all of their son's needs. She does not like to visit with them because of this.*

With the first example, it would have been impossible to define the problem or come up with a solution. When the problem situation was clearly defined, it was easier to get a picture of the true problem.

Now I would like you to try your hand at clearly defining terms and problems. I have taken the liberty of rewriting Donna's story in such a way that it is difficult to figure out what her problem is. This new version is re-

corded on the handout that I will pass out to you now (pass out Handout #3, Appendix B-5). Pay close attention to those words and passages that are in italics. After I finish reading this aloud, I would like you to choose a partner to work with. Together, you and your partner will work on clearing up all of the confusion. Redefine all the words and situations that are italicized in the handout. You will find the answers in the original version of Donna's story that I passed out first. After you are finished, we will come together as a group and talk about the exercise.

Review of Handout #2 (Appendix B-5): Version Two of Donna's Story

Donna doesn't *hang out* much anymore. She just does her *daily stuff.* A *couple* times a week she goes to meetings. But that's it. She's worried about *getting strung out* again and *missing* her kids. Donna just feels kind of *yucky.* She doesn't want help from her group because she's not into that *'God stuff.'*

Directions: Give the women some time to work. Then ask the following questions.

- When reading Version Two of Donna's Story, could you get a clear picture of what was going on with her? Why not?

- Would someone like to begin redefining the words that were in italics? (Go through all of the words.) Record these on the blackboard.

- It is very important to get a clear picture of word definitions and problem situations. When problems are fuzzy, we need to seek more information. If we did not have the first version of Donna's story to refer to, what are some of ways we could have used to get more information about Donna's problem? [Example: a) ask Donna to clearly define terms she used, b) find out what kind of meetings Donna attends.] Record these on the blackboard.

- In your own life, can you think of a time when gathering more information would have been helpful in defining a problem? Why?

■ Closure of the Session (approximate time: 5 minutes)

    a. Summary

    b. Homework assignment

Summary: Briefly summarize the major points covered in the body of Session 3 (#2 through #4). Ask members if they have any questions.

Homework Assignment: Ask members to continue keeping an informal journal. Have the women look over past entries for fuzzy terms and then redefine those terms in a clear manner. In addition to identifying problems, they should begin to practice problem definition in their journal entries.

★ Remind members of the time and day of the next meeting.

Session Overview

Concept: Systematic Definition

- Dissect the problem into manageable concrete units, operationally defining each unit.
- Thorough exploration of all aspects of the problem.
    a. Differentiate important from unimportant information.
    b. Establish appropriate goals.
    c. Explore subproblems and potential conflicts.
- Gather additional information, if necessary.
- Clearly state the problem.

Session Objectives

- The client will be able to establish appropriate goals through identification of behavioral objectives (desired outcomes) and desired reinforcement.
- The client will be able to identify possible obstacles and conflicts with established goals.
- The client will be able to integrate the information gathered in Step 1 and Step 2 of the problem-solving model into a concise problem statement.

Session Format

1. Introduction
    a. Review of Session 3
    b. Overview of Session 4
2. Goal setting
    a. Identifying goals
3. Exploring subproblems
    a. Obstacles
    b. Conflicts with other self-selected goals
    c. Conflicts with the goals of other people
4. Stating the problem
    a. Integrating information
5. Closure of the session

a. Summary

b. Homework assignment

Materials Needed

- Lecture notes
- Blackboard, chalk and eraser, or large sheets of paper, markers, and tacks
- Handout #2 and #4 (Appendix B-5)
- Game cards (Appendix A-3)
- Overhead #2 (Appendix C)

■ Introduction (approximate time: 10 minutes)

Review: Summarize the major points covered in Session 3. You may use the overview of the session below for this purpose.

Session 3 Review

2. Transitioning from problem identification to problem definition.

    a. Differences between identification and definition.

    b. How the two components work together.

3. Making problems more manageable: breaking them down into concrete parts.

    a. Identifying relevant information: external and internal events.

    b. Exploring background information.

4. Learning to clarify problems.

    a. Operationally defining terms.

    b. Recognizing an impasse: when to seek more information.

Ask group members if they have any questions or comments. Solicit any input they may have about the homework assignment. How did the journal work for them? How did changing fuzzy terms prove helpful?

Overview: Review the major points that will be covered in this session. Emphasize that this session will concentrate on problems in general and in detail, and on setting goals that will allow for the solution of these problems.

■ Goal Setting (approximate time: 20 minutes)

a. Identifying general goals

Materials Needed

- Lecture notes
- Blackboard, chalk and eraser, or large sheets of paper, markers, and tacks
- Handout #2 (Appendix B-5)

Lecture and Group Exercise Format: A brief lecture concerning the importance of goal setting should be presented to the group. A sample lecture covering the major points to be made is provided below. You may use this lecture verbatim or you may use your own words, in which case, be sure to cover the major content and themes that are contained in the sample lecture. Following your lecture, the group should be given the opportunity to work together in formulating their goals by using Session 3, "Donna's Story: Version One" (Handout #2, Appendix B-5). Directions for this follow the sample lecture.

Sample Lecture: *Now that we have learned to specifically define our problems, we will explore how to identify goals for dealing with them. In doing so we need to make sure that the goals we choose fit our problems, and also that our goals are clearly defined. This will help us to think of other solutions to them later on.*

What would happen if our goals did not fit our problems? Or, what would happen if our goals were too fuzzy? Or, even worse, what would happen if we had no goals at all? Chances are that we would have limited or no success in solving our problems. Thus, if we expect to find solutions that satisfy us, we will have to give thought as to what should be our goals.

After defining each problem situation, you should answer two questions:

a. What are some things that might make your situation better?

b. What do you want to see happen in terms of results or outcomes?

Answers to these questions will help you to create goals that will fit your problem and bring you closer to a possible solution. Using Donna's Story from our last session, let's practice asking these questions for Donna and identify some goals for her. It sounded as though she could use our help. In order to refresh our memory, I will pass the handout back to you and read the story aloud.

Lesson Plan

Directions: After reading the problem situation aloud to the group, help them to recall the various aspects of Donna's problem (important information: external and internal). A copy of these is provided below. Using these aspects, have them generate a list of general goals that might help Donna with her problem. Be sure that the group deals only with general goals. Use the questions emphasized in the lecture. (What are some things that might make Donna's situation better? and What do I want to see happen in terms of results or outcomes?) Record their responses on the blackboard. Have each member explain why she chose a particular goal for Donna. Encourage the group to interact in this process. Sample lists of important information and general goals follow:

Important Information

External:

— All of Donna's time is spent in structured situations: home, work, and meetings.

— Donna spends minimum time socializing.

— Much of Donna's time is spent working.

— Donna does not have any play time away from responsibilities.

— Donna is avoiding people for various reasons.

— Donna's primary interactions are with her two children.

Internal:

— Donna is tired, scared, and lonely.

— She is afraid of losing her children.

— Religion and God are subjects that Donna is uncomfortable with.

Sample List of Goals

— Develop a new support system.

— Learn time-management skills.

— Learn to play again.

— Work on spirituality issues.

— Get some help with domestic duties.

■ Exploring Subproblems (approximate time: 40 minutes)

    a.   Obstacles

    b.   Conflicts with other self-selected goals

    c.   Conflicts with the goals of other people

Materials Needed

- Lecture notes
- Game cards (Appendix A-3)

Lecture and Group Game Format: Identification of potential subproblems to major problems is one component of the problem-solving model that can further clarify a problem situation and enhance the production of alternatives. A sample lecture covering the major points outlined above has been provided for you. You may use the lecture verbatim or you may use your own words to convey the information. If you choose to use your own words, be sure to cover the major content and themes that are contained in the sample lecture.

Following the lecture, group members should participate in a game that is designed to help them identify subproblems and differentiate between obstacles and conflicts. There are two problem situations used in the game. Each problem situation has a set of 'Sorry!' cards that is used with it. Encouraging members to respond, interact, and challenge one another is essential to the success of this exercise.

Sample Lecture: *After you have identified some general goals for your problem situation, you will need to investigate what we call "subproblems." Subproblems come in two forms, obstacles or conflicts. Obstacles are anything that might get in the way of you accomplishing your goals. For example, you may lack the resources needed to reach your goal. If you need transportation and have none, that is an obstacle. In contrast, conflicts come about because you or someone else, have desires that are in competition with your new goal. For example, you may wish to enjoy the early morning hours by getting outdoors. However, your new goal conflicts with another one of your goals, always having an adult at home to supervise your children. If you went out, there would be nobody to watch the children. Your two goals are in conflict with one another.*

Sometimes, what appears to be an obstacle or a conflict, upon closer inspection is really not one at all. At other times a real obstacle or conflict can be, in some way, overcome. In either case, it is better to explore poten-

tial obstacles and conflicts before going ahead with solutions. Because of them, you may need to go back and collect more information to clear up any questions that come up. This will save you time. Knowing what your subproblems are will help you later on when you are creating a list of possible solutions and when you must decide among those solutions.

We are going to practice identifying potential obstacles and conflicts using a game format. I need one person who is willing to be the owner of a problem. The rest of the group members will present you with potential obstacles and conflicts which may or may not get in the way of your goal. It will be your job to decide if there is a real obstacle or conflict and explain your decision to the group. Why did you or why didn't you think that there was an obstacle or conflict? The group will then vote on your decision, adding any thoughts or ideas they might have. We have two practice situations to work with. Who would like to volunteer to be the owner of the first problem?

Use game cards here (Appendix A-3).

Directions:
a. Give the volunteer a problem card and ask her to read it aloud to the group.
b. Ask a group member to choose one "Sorry!" (Appendix A-3) card to read aloud.
c. The volunteer should then respond by deciding if there is a potential conflict, obstacle, or neither with regard to the stated goal. She should justify her answer.
d. Using the "Vote" cards (Appendix A-4), ask each member is to cast a vote as to whether she agrees or disagrees with the volunteer. They should justify their responses. "Thumbs Up" for agree, "thumbs down" for disagree.
e. Another member should then be asked to choose a "Sorry!" card (Appendix A-3). Follow the same process as above until all of the "Sorry!" cards have been used.

- **Stating the Problem (approximate time: 15 minutes)**
    a. Integrating information

Materials Needed

Lecture notes

✏ Handout #4 (Appendix B-5)

✏ Overhead #2 (Appendix C)

Lecture and Modeling Format: This section is designed to help group members use what they have learned to make a clear problem statement. A clear problem statement will later facilitate their production of alternatives. A sample lecture, that includes the use of modeling, has been provided for this purpose. Again, you may use the lecture verbatim or you may use your own words. If you choose to use your own words, be careful to cover the major content and themes that are contained in the sample lecture. Distribute Handout #4 (Appendix B-5) and use it as a visual aid during the presentation.

Sample Lecture: *We have done a good deal of work thus far in identifying and defining various parts of problem situations. The handout shows us all of the major areas we have covered. Before we move on to search for solutions, we have one final task. We each need to state the problem. This should be done by using the information you have already gathered in the steps shown in the handout. Because we have done all the leg work, stating the problem is made simple. All you have to do is put the information together. I will show you how this can be done by using the last problem situation in the game we just played.*

📄 Use Overhead #2 (Appendix C).

We will use the handout to work through the problem.

a. *The problem has already been identified. We know that (name of the volunteer) owns the problem. The major issue appears to be the need to manage stress in a healthier way. The problem owner has managed to stop and think. She has not resorted to her old way of coping with her problem. She has not used drugs. Good for her.*

b. *Important information would include: she is home alone, it does not appear as though she has any means of support available to her during the day, she feels she has a good deal of work to do each day (external); she feels overwhelmed, anxious, and tense, she wants help, she wants to stay clean (internal).*

To clear up terms or words used, we may want to ask her to tell us what she means when she says she feels overwhelmed, tense, or anxious. These words may mean different things for her depending on her circumstances. For example, "overwhelmed" in this case may mean that she never gets all of the work done that she has planned for herself in a day. She feels like she is behind and will never catch up.

c. Her stated goal was to get help during the day. She wants help staying sober and she wants to manage her stress better. Her subproblems may include: little support from important family members, no transportation, and no direct 12-step support system available during the day.

Using this information, I now can state her problem. Our problem person needs help in learning new ways to manage her stress during the day. She would like a balance between the amount of time she has and the amount of work she can accomplish during that time. She would also like some kind of support system available to her during the day to maintain her sobriety.

The problem is stated in such a way that it becomes clear that there are two areas for which we need solutions: learning to manage stress and establishing a support system during the day. All the information available was condensed into one manageable unit. Keep in mind that there is no one perfect way to state a problem. What we are trying to do is focus on the core issues and goals.

Problem statements should be as clear and as specific as possible. Our purpose is to cut down on confusion and give direction to our problem solving. In this way, we will have a better picture of what we will need to do. Our problem then won't look so overwhelming. By using the steps that we have been working on, our problems will be more manageable. We will be giving ourselves an opportunity to find solutions that work best for us.

■ Closure of the Session (approximate time: 5 minutes)

   a. Summary
   b. Homework assignment

Summary: Briefly summarize the major points covered in this session and then follow-up by asking the group if they have any questions.

Homework Assignment: For the next session, the group should be prepared to practice identifying, defining, and stating a problem. Ask that each member practice using these skills in their journal until the next session. These skills will then be tied into Step 3 of the problem-solving model: production of alternatives.

★ Remind members of the time and day of the next meeting.

Session Overview

Concept: Production of Alternatives
- Brainstorm a number of alternative solutions to problems.

Session Objectives
- The client will be able to distinguish between general goals and the specific alternative solutions selected for achieving goals.
- The client will be able to put into practice four rules of brainstorming when generating alternative solutions.

Session Format
1. Introduction
    a. Review of Session 4
    b. Overview of Session 5
2. Producing alternatives
    a. Clarity as an important factor
    b. The difference between general goals and alternative solutions.
3. Four rules of brainstorming
    a. Openness
    b. Creativity
    c. Quantity
    d. Improvement
4. Closure of the session
    a. Summary
    b. Homework assignment

Materials Needed
- Lecture notes
- Blackboard, chalk and eraser, or large sheets of paper, markers, and tacks
- Illustration #1 (Appendix D)
- Handouts #2 and #5 (Appendix B-5)

■ Introduction (approximate time: 10 minutes)

Review: Summarize the major points covered in Session 4. You may use the overview of the session below for this purpose.

Session 4 Review

2. Goal setting
   a. Identifying general goals
3. Exploring subproblems
   a. Obstacles
   b. Conflicts with other self-selected goals
   c. Conflicts with the goals of other people
4. Stating the problem
   a. Integrating information

Ask the group if they have any questions or comments. Solicit any input they may have about the homework assignment. How did the journal work for them? Are they getting a clearer picture of the problem situations they identify for themselves?

Overview: Review the major points that will be covered in Session 5. You may use the overview of the session for this purpose. Learning Step 3 of the problem-solving model, Production of Alternatives, is the goal for this lesson.

■ Producing Alternatives (approximate time: 30 minutes)

   a. Clarity as an important factor
   b. The difference between general goals and alternative solutions

Materials Needed

- Lecture notes
- Blackboard, chalk and eraser, or large sheets of paper, markers, and tacks
- Illustration #1 (Appendix D)

Lecture and Group Exercise: A brief lecture presentation should be used to introduce the concepts. A sample lecture is provided below for this purpose. You may use the lecture verbatim or you may use your own words. If you choose to use your own words, be careful to cover the major content and themes that are contained in the sample lecture. Following your lecture, the group should engage in an exercise designed to assist them in distinguishing between their goals and the alternatives they propose to solve their problems. Illustration #1 provides a visual aid for this concept.

Sample Lecture: *We have learned that it is important to be clear about what we mean. In Step 3 of the problem-solving model, Producing Alternatives, clearness is essential. Obviously, it would be difficult to make a reasonable choice among our proposed solutions if we did not understand what was involved in each suggested solution. For example, you and your friend find yourselves in a very uncomfortable situation on a bus with several men bothering you. You will want to restore your sense of comfort. Your friend nudges you and whispers "let's do something about this now." What does this mean? Her statement might mean any number of things. It could mean getting off of the bus at the next stop and phoning home for a ride. She might mean asking the bus driver to talk to the men. Your friend might also mean that she is about to make an assertive request directly to the men who are bothering you.*

As we can see by this example, when a planned solution is not made clear a lot of confusion and mistakes can result. Restated, it is important for you to make things clear and definite when you try to solve a problem.

📄 Distribute Illustration #1 (Appendix D) at this point.

It has already been noted that a general goal is simply a statement about a desired outcome—to have the problem solved. Put another way, a goal is broad and may be thought of as an umbrella. Alternative solutions, on the other hand, are what I mean as the variety of approaches one may consider in reaching a goal. They fit under the umbrella.

Consider for a moment the illustration I have just handed you. Now imagine that you are a student who is not doing well in school. Your goal (desired outcome) is to improve your grades. You then consider alternatives for achieving your goal. You might think about improving your grades by studying in the morning when you are refreshed rather than at night when you are tired. Or, you might consider improving your grades by taking notes in class or on the written assignments you have done and then reviewing them regularly. Perhaps a considered solution is to improve your eating habits. Your goal is to improve your grades. It is the umbrella. Changing your study time, taking notes, or changing eating habits are all possible solutions to your problem of low grades. Restated once

Lesson Plan

again, after we choose a general goal that fits our problem situation best, we then consider possible solutions for achieving that goal.

Now we will practice identifying goals for ourselves and some possible solutions or plans for achieving them. Here is a brief sample problem.

Exercise Directions: Read aloud "Sue's Problem" and then ask the group to identify Sue's two most obvious goals. Draw a diagram similar to the one that follows on an easel or blackboard to record her goals. After this is completed, ask the group to suggest some possible solutions that would fit under each of the goals. Record these on the blackboard. After completing the exercise, again discuss the difference between a general goal and alternative solutions. Then ask how the goals and proposed solutions are relevant to each other.

Sue's Problem: Sue is unhappy with her life and would like to improve it. She has had several lapses in sobriety recently and is not getting along well with the people she cares about.

Sue's Goals: Sue has identified two general goals that may be a way of improving her life. One is to stay sober. The other is to improve her relationships with others.

Diagramming Sue's Goals and Proposed Solutions

Goal	Possible Alternative Solutions
• Stay sober	• Attend 12-step meeting • Call for support • Don't use • Work on issues
• Improve relationships	• Be honest • Make amends for past behavior • Be assertive not aggressive • Put aside time for kids

Session 5	47

- **Four Rules of Brainstorming (approximate time: 45 minutes)**
    1. Openness
    2. Creativity
    3. Quantity
    4. Improvement

Materials Needed

- Lecture notes
- Blackboard, chalk and eraser, or large sheets of paper, markers, and tacks
- Handouts #2 and #5 (Appendix B-5)

Lecture and Group Exercise Format: A brief lecture presentation should be used to introduce the four concepts outlined above. A sample lecture is provided below that you may use. If you use your own words, be sure to cover the major content and themes that are contained in the sample lecture. (Before the presentation, distribute Handout #5 (Appendix B-5) to each member.) After your lecture engage the group in an exercise designed to assist them in learning to apply brainstorming rules to the production of alternative solutions.

Sample Lecture: *We have been talking about producing alternative solutions for problem situations. Having a number of solutions to choose from improves our chances of selecting the best solution or combination of solutions. For any given goal, we will need to produce a number of solutions before deciding which solution best fits our goal for the problem situation.*

To be effective we need a road map to follow, i.e., some guidelines that will help us to create the solutions we need. The approach we will use is called "brainstorming."

Effective brainstorming usually employs four basic rules. On the handout I've given out are key words that label these rules for effective brainstorming. I use these key words to remind myself of the rules or guidelines.

*Let's look at the first word: "**Openness.**" Rule #1 of brainstorming is that we must remain open to each and every alternative. When brainstorming, judgment, and criticism should be withheld. We will judge each solution later. Until then, we should suspend judgment.*

*The next word listed on our handout is **"Creativity."** Rule #2 of brainstorming is to be original, and wild; to be the first one on our block to come up with a valuable solution. Creativity, in other words, is not only welcome, it is desired.*

*Rule #3 is represented by the word **"Quantity."** When we are brainstorming we need to consider as many solutions to our problem as possible. The more solutions we can come up with, the better.*

*The last word listed on the handout is **"Improvement."** Rule #4 requires that we attempt to improve upon the solutions we have considered. We may suggest a way to make someone else's idea better, or we may combine several ideas into one great idea. Either way, what we are looking for is improvement.*

Now let's try our hand at brainstorming. We will pick on Donna one last time.

Distribute Handout # 2 (Appendix B-5) at this point.

After I am finished reading Donna's problem situation, I will briefly review some of the past work we have done with her problem. Together we will write out a problem statement and then choose one goal to work on. Using the brainstorming approach I have just described, we will then practice coming up with solutions that might help Donna meet her goal. Remember that clearly defined solutions will help us greatly.

Donna's Story

Directions: Read Donna's problem situation aloud to the group. After you finish reading, review the section labeled, "Important Information," and then ask the group to create a problem statement. Write the problem statement on the blackboard. A sample problem statement is provided for this purpose. Finally, review the "Sample List of Goals" and ask the group to choose a goal to work on. Using the brainstorming rules, have the members produce alternative solutions. Throughout the exercise encourage adherence to brainstorming rules. Record the alternative solutions they produce on the blackboard. Give specific positive reinforcement for the brainstorming rules they apply (such as creativity or improvement). Model desired behavior by occasionally adding an alternative solution to the group's list. State which rule(s) you used in generating the alternative.

A minimum of 10 to 15 alternatives should be produced. Repeat the above directions with a second goal.

Important Information

External:

— All of Donna's time is spent in structured situations: home, work, and meetings.

— Donna spends minimum time socializing.

— Donna is avoiding people for various reasons.

Internal:

— Donna is tired, scared, and lonely.

— She is afraid of losing her children.

— Religion and God are subjects that Donna is uncomfortable with.

Sample Problem Statement

Donna is not happy with the way things are in her life right now. She wants to have a little more energy and not be so lonely.

Sample List of Goals

— Develop a new support system.

— Learn to play again.

— Understand the difference between religion and spirituality.

■ Closure of the Session (approximate time: 5 minutes)

    a. Summary

    b. Homework assignment

Summary: Briefly summarize the major points covered in the body of Session 5. Ask members if there are any questions.

Homework Assignment: Ask everyone to continue writing in their journals. Have the women look over their past entries and practice the brainstorming skills on their problems—the ones they have already identified and defined.

★ Remind members of the place, time, and day of the next meeting.

Session Overview

Concept: Production of Alternatives
- Brainstorm a number of alternative solutions.

Concept: Evaluation of Alternatives and Decision
- Exploration of the potential outcomes of alternatives.
- Gather additional information, if necessary.
- Arrange alternative solutions in a hierarchy according to perceived effectiveness.
- Choose an alternative.

Session Objectives
- The client will be able to eliminate obviously inferior alternative solutions.
- The client will be able to evaluate remaining alternative solutions by exploring potential outcomes and consequences of each alternative.
- Using all the information gathered, the client will be able to rank alternative solutions in a hierarchy of most to least desirable.
- The client will be able to choose one alternative solution to implement.

Session Format
1. Introduction
   a. Review of Session 5
   b. Overview of Session 6
2. Producing alternatives through brainstorming
3. Evaluating alternatives and making a decision
   a. Screening alternatives
   b. Exploring possible outcomes
   c. Ranking alternatives
   d. Making a decision
4. Integrating Step 3 and Step 4 of the problem-solving model
5. Closure of the session

Session 6

a. Summary
b. Homework Assignment

Materials Needed

- Lecture notes
- Blackboard, chalk and eraser, or large sheets of paper, markers, and tacks
- Handout #5 (Appendix B-5) for review of Session 5
- Overhead #3 (Appendix C) for review of Session 5
- Handout #6 (Appendix B-5)
- Voting cards (Appendix A-4)

■ Introduction (approximate time: 10 minutes)

Review: Summarize the major points covered in Session 5. You may use the overview of the session for this purpose.

Session 5 Review

2. Producing alternatives
   a. The difference between general goals and alternative solutions
   b. Clarity as an important factor
3. The four rules of brainstorming
   a. Openness
   b. Creativity
   c. Quantity
   d. Improvement

Ask if anyone has any questions or comments. Solicit any input they may have about the homework assignment. How did the journal work for them? Were they able to successfully apply all of the brainstorming rules?

Overview: Summarize the major points that will be covered in this session. You may use the format above for this purpose.

Session 6 53

■ Producing Alternatives through Brainstorming (approximate time: 25 minutes)

Materials Needed

- Lecture notes
- Blackboard, chalk and eraser, or large sheets of paper, markers, and tacks
- Handout #5 (Appendix B-5)
- Overhead #3 (Appendix C)

Lecture and Group Exercise: A brief lecture presentation should be used to review brainstorming rules presented in Session 5. A sample lecture is provided below for this purpose. You may use the lecture verbatim or you may use your own words. If you choose to use your own words, be careful to cover the major content and themes that are contained in the sample lecture.

Distribute Handout #5 (Appendix B-5).

Following the presentation, a group exercise should be used to help members master the skill of brainstorming alternative solutions. Display Overhead #3 (Appendix C) and read the problem situation aloud. Ask everyone to produce alternative solutions. Again, encourage the group to adhere to the rules for brainstorming. Record their solutions on the blackboard. Continue to give positive reinforcement for the rules they apply (i.e., creativity or improvement). Model desired behavior by occasionally adding an alternative solution to the group's list. State which rule(s) you used in producing the alternative.

A minimum of 10 to 15 alternatives should be produced.

Sample Lecture: *During our last session we learned the four basic rules of brainstorming. Let's review those one more time. If you recall, we needed a road map to produce solutions. We used brainstorming as a guide to discovering alternative solutions to our problem situations. The four basic rules of brainstorming are as follows:*

Rule #1: Openness

Remain open to each and every alternative. When brainstorming, judgment and criticism are withheld. No opinions please.

Lesson Plan

Rule #2: Creativity

Be original, be wild, don't be afraid to be different. Creativity is not only welcomed, it is desired.

Rule #3: Quantity

Produce as many alternative solutions as possible. The more alternatives we can generate, the better it is.

Rule #4: Improvement

Improve upon the alternatives that are produced. Make them better. We can suggest a way to make someone else's idea better or we can combine several ideas into one great idea.

Now that we have reviewed the rules, let's practice producing some solutions. After we have finished, we will learn to evaluate each of the alternatives. Listen to the following problem situation.

Use Overhead #3 (Appendix C).

Problem Situation: Stacey hates to get her mail. It seems like the overdue notices come everyday. She has so many bills that she has lost track of how much she owes and to whom. Her landlord is threatening to evict her and last week the phone service was shut off.

It's not that Stacey doesn't earn a good salary. She does. But Stacey sometimes gets depressed and wants to feel better. A shopping trip usually can pull her right up out of her depression. Shopping works really well until it is over. Then Stacey feels guilty, ashamed, and more depressed than ever. She knows she can't afford her buying sprees. Sometimes Stacey thinks that her money problem is as bad as her drinking problem used to be.

General Goals (choose one): (1) Stacey's immediate problem is a financial one. She would like to find a way to pay off her bills and still have enough money to live on every month; (2) Stacey would also like to learn another way to deal with her depression.

▪ Evaluating Alternatives and Making a Decision (approximate time: 20 minutes)

    a. Screening alternatives

    b. Exploring possible outcomes

    c. Ranking alternatives

    d.   Making a decision

Materials Needed

- Lecture Notes
- Blackboard, chalk and eraser, or large sheets of paper, markers and tacks
- Handout #6 (Appendix B-5)

Lecture Format: A lecture presentation should be used to present Step 4 of the problem-solving model, *Evaluation of Alternatives and Decisions*. A sample lecture has been provided for this purpose. You may use the lecture verbatim or you can use your own words to convey the information. If you choose to use your own words, be careful to cover the major content and themes that are contained in the sample lecture.

Distribute Handout #6 (Appendix B-5).

The lecture content follows along with the outline presented in Handout #6.

Sample Lecture: *We have just practiced brainstorming alternatives. This was done by keeping in mind the goals for a problem situation. There are many alternative solutions to any problem. What concerns us most is picking the solution that will meet our goals and, therefore, work best for us in a given situation. We are about to learn a very organized and effective way to evaluate the alternatives available to us. The handout I have just given you contains an outline of the approach we will use.*

Let's look at #1 Select Out Inferior Alternatives. This is the first step of the evaluation process. When done correctly, screening can save us a lot of time. What we want to do at this step is to get rid of or eliminate any alternative that is obviously inferior. That means we will scratch off our list any solution that is sure to bring about negative consequences. For example, we would want to eliminate any alternative that would bring physical harm to ourselves or another person.

After we have screened our list of alternatives and eliminated very poor ones, we can begin to evaluate the alternatives that are left. Look at #2 Exploring Potential Outcomes, on your handout. As you can see, there are several things to consider: areas the consequences can occur—individual and public, the time frame the consequences can take place—immediate and future, rating the consequence—positive, neutral, or negative, and finally the possibility that the consequence will occur at all—very likely, likely, or unlikely. For each alternative, we need to think about each of the these factors. If things are a bit unclear, we will need to go back and gather more information about each consequence and the factors involved. I will use an example to illustrate these factors.

Remember Donna? How can we forget Donna. One goal for Donna would be to develop a new group of friends. Since staying sober is important to her, Donna thinks that she could make friends by spending more time with 12-step members after the meeting. This is one alternative. Now let's look at the factors we were just discussing.

The Consequences that Can Occur

Individual: In this area we want to look at Donna's feelings, needs, and desires. How will spending more time with 12-step members after the meeting affect her personally? Perhaps she won't be lonely any more.

Public: Consider the impact the alternative will have on other people in Donna's life, and consider other people's reaction to Donna. How will spending more time with 12-step members after the meeting affect her and others socially? Perhaps her parents will disapprove because they don't want to believe she has a drinking problem. Or perhaps there are 12-step members who would be grateful to have a new friend.

Time Frame in Which the Consequences Can Take Place

Immediate: Right now, how will spending more time with 12-step members after the meeting affect Donna? Perhaps she will get some relief from her loneliness.

Future: Looking ahead, how will spending more time with 12-step members after the meeting affect Donna? She could establish several long term satisfying relationships.

Rating the consequence: positive, neutral, or negative. In evaluating the alternative of spending more time with 12-step members after the meeting, Donna thought one consequence might be that she would be less lonely. In light of her goal, to make new friends, Donna would rate this consequence as positive.

Possibility that the consequence will occur at all: very likely, likely, or unlikely. This is the last factor Donna must consider. In evaluating the alternative, Donna thought one consequence might be that she would be less lonely. She believes that this consequence is likely to occur.

Now look at #3, Rank the Alternatives. We have gathered all the important information we need on each alternative. We are now able to rank the alternatives according to their attractiveness. In other words, we will rate them according to how well we think they will meet our goals. The alternative that we believe will succeed best in meeting our goals is placed at the top of the list. The alternative that appears to be least able to meet our goals will be put at the bottom of the list. In the process of ranking alternatives, it is important to consider all of the information that has been gathered about each alternative.

Finally we come to #4, Make a Decision. It is time to make a choice. Now is the moment that we will either choose one alternative or a set of alternatives. Keeping the goals we have in mind for the problem situation, we make our choice . . . and then try it out.

■ Integrating Step 3 and Step 4 of the Problem-Solving Model (approximate time: 30 minutes)

Materials Needed

- Lecture notes
- Blackboard, chalk and eraser, or large sheets of paper, marker and tacks
- Handout #6 (Appendix B-5)
- Voting Cards (Appendix A-4)

Group Exercise Format: Using the general strategies generated for the Problem Situation (Stacey) in Part 2 of this session, assist group members in learning to apply the four steps of the evaluation process just taught in Part 3. Handout #6 should be used as a direct guide in the evaluation of alternatives. Guide the group through each step and record their responses on the blackboard. Use the Vote Cards (Appendix A-4) in the first step of the evaluation process. Ask members to hold their cards up to vote for which alternatives they want to retain (thumbs up) and which alternatives they want to screen out (thumbs down). Each member should then give a rationale for their vote.

You will probably want to use only two or three of the alternatives to evaluate due to time limitations. In Session 7, the group will have the opportunity to work through the entire process using one problem situation.

- **Closure of the Session (approximate time: 5 minutes)**
    a. Summary
    b. Homework assignment

Summary: Briefly summarize the major points covered in the body of Session 6 (#2 through #4). Ask members if they have any questions.

Homework Assignment: Ask members to continue writing in their journals. Have the women look over their past entries and practice the brainstorming skills on problems they have already identified and defined. In addition, they should practice evaluating the alternatives they have generated.

★ Remind members of the place, time, and day of the next meeting.

Session Overview

Concept: Familiarization
- Acknowledgment and acceptance that problem situations are a common occurrence in daily living.
- Recognition and identification of problem situations as they occur.
- Restraint of automatic responses to problem situations.

Concept: Systematic Definition
- Dissect the problem into manageable concrete units, operationally defining each unit.
- Through exploration of all aspects of the problem:
    a. differentiate important from unimportant information;
    b. establish appropriate goals;
    c. explore subproblems and potential conflicts.
- Gather additional information, if necessary.
- Clearly state the problem.

Concept: Production of Alternatives
- Brainstorm a number of alternative solutions.

Concept: Evaluation of Alternatives and Decision
- Exploration of the potential outcomes of alternatives.
- Gather additional information, if necessary.
- Arrange alternative solutions in a hierarchy according to perceived effectiveness.
- Choose an alternative.

Session Objectives
- Using several sample problems, the client will be able to integrate information taught in Steps 1 through 4 of the problem-solving model and properly sequence problem-solving skills.

Session Format
1. Introduction

Session 7

        a. Review of Session 6
        b. Overview of Session 7
    2. Integrating Steps 1 through 3 of the problem-solving model.
    3. Closure of the session
        a. Summary
        b. Homework assignment

Materials Needed

- Lecture notes
- Blackboard, chalk and eraseer, or large sheets of paper, markers, and tacks
- Handouts #5 & #7 (Appendix B-5)
- Role play cards (Appendix A-2)
- Vote cards (Appendix A-4)

■ Introduction (approximate time: 10 minutes)

Review: Summarize the major points covered in Session 6. You can use the overview of the session provided below for this purpose.

Session 6 Review

    2. Review of brainstorming rules
        a. Producing alternative solutions
    3. Evaluating alternatives and making a decision
        a. Screening alternatives
        b. Exploring possible outcomes
        c. Ranking alternatives
        d. Making a decision
    4. Integrating Step 3 and Step 4 of the problem-solving model.

Ask if anyone has any questions or comments. Solicit any input they may have about the homework assignment. How did the journal work for them? Were they able to successfully apply all of the brainstorming rules and evaluate each alternative to their problem situation?

Overview: During today's session, the group will practice skills they have learned from the first four steps of the model.

- **Integrating Steps 1 through 4 of the Problem-Solving Model (approximate time: 75 minutes)**

Materials Needed

- Lecture notes
- Blackboard, chalk and eraser, or large sheets of paper, markers, and tacks
- Handout #5 & #7 (Appendix B-5)
- Role play cards (Appendix A-2)
- Vote cards (Appendix A-4)

Lecture and Group Exercise Format: A brief lecture presentation will be used to introduce the practice exercise presented in Session 7. A sample lecture has been provided for this purpose. You may use the lecture verbatim or you can use your own words to convey the information. If you choose to use your own words, be careful to cover the major content and themes that are contained in the sample lecture. After the presentation, distribute Handout #5 (Appendix B-5) and Handout #7 (Appendix B-5) to each member. These two handouts will act as a guide and visual prompt during the exercise. The purpose of the exercise is to assist members with integration and mastery of the skills in Steps 1 through 4 of the problem-solving model. Each of the two role-play cards provided for this session contain a problem situation. Ask for two volunteers from the group who are willing to role play each of the problem situations. Assist them if necessary.

After each role play, ask the group members to identify and define the problem, using Handout #7 (Appendix B-5) as a guide. Brainstorming alternative solutions should be followed by evaluation of the alternatives. Again, use Handout #5 and #7 (Appendix B-5) as a guide. Vote Cards should be used during both the screening and decision-making steps. Ask the members to hold their cards up to vote for which alternatives they want (thumbs up) and which alternatives they do not want (thumbs down). Each member should give a rationale for their vote.

📄 Distribute Handouts #5 and #7 (Appendix B-5).

Record the responses generated by the group on the blackboard. Continue to give specific positive reinforcement for effort and the rules that they are applying. Model desired behavior making sure to verbalize

Lesson Plan

your thought processes. Due to time constraints, the group may not be able to finish its work on the second role play. If this is the case, allow the group to do as much work as possible.

Before getting started, spend approximately 10 minutes helping the women visualize themselves as effective problem solvers. The visualization exercise used previously is provided below for this purpose.

Visualization Exercise

Directions: Now I want to invite everybody to see themselves as effective problem solvers by using our visualization exercise. Again, all you have to do is follow my directions. Are you ready? First, I want you to get as comfortable as possible. Take your shoes off if that helps. . . . Good. Now close your eyes, here we go.

Exercise: *Keeping your eyes closed, I want you to take a few deep breaths . . . slowly breathe in . . . and . . . breathe out . . . inhale . . . exhale. Good. With each breath you feel yourself becoming more and more relaxed . . . more and more calm . . . inhale . . . exhale. That's right. . . . Nothing can disturb your sense of peace and . . . tranquility . . . nothing can bother you . . . there are no pressing matters . . . nothing that needs your attention . . . you are free to relax . . . and enjoy the calm peacefulness . . . with each passing moment . . . you find yourself . . . more and more . . . relaxed. Tension is leaving your body . . . slowly draining away . . . with each breath you feel more and more comfortable . . . more calm. Time loses all meaning for you . . . it no longer matters . . . as you feel the peacefulness gently come over you. You are now entering a different world . . . the road is easy to travel . . . because you feel . . . calm . . . relaxed . . . and successful in the new world. Let your mind take you there . . . your special place where you feel peace and serenity surround you . . . hugging your body . . . your very being. Take a look around you and notice . . . the sights . . . the smells . . . and the sounds. What a wonderful place this is . . . so quiet and peaceful. Enjoy the relaxing atmosphere of your special place . . . in your special place . . . you can deal with anything that happens . . . relaxed . . . confident . . . calm . . . experience the good feelings of success and mastery . . . nothing is impossible . . . you can take care of whatever comes your way . . . when you see a problem coming . . . you are . . . very calm . . . calm and peaceful . . . confident that you can take care of the problem. And you do . . . it feels good to take care of things and move on . . . skilled . . . confident . . . sure of yourself. You did so well . . . you can feel good about your abilities . . . relaxed . . . successful. . . . And now its time to leave your special place . . . you can come back whenever you want . . .*

you can bring back the good feelings you had in your special place . . . peacefulness . . . strength . . . confidence . . . success. Slowly come back . . . as you become more and more aware of your breathing . . . once again . . . come back. At the count of five . . . I want you to open your eyes . . . one . . . two . . . three . . . four . . . five . . . now open your eyes.

Directions: Give the group members a few moments to re-orient themselves. Invite any of the members who would like to comment on their experience to share with the group and then proceed with the lecture below.

Sample Lecture: *We are finally going to get a chance to put together everything we have learned thus far. I will pass around two handouts that will help us with today's exercise. One will look familiar. It has the four key words for the brainstorming rules. The other handout has an overview of the problem-solving model we have learned so far. After we role play a problem situation, we can use these two handouts as guides in the problem-solving process. We will work through four steps of the problem-solving model: identifying the problem, defining the problem, producing alternatives and finally, evaluating them and making a decision. Let's get started.*

Materials Needed

- Use Role-Play Cards here (Appendix A-2)
- Copies of Handouts #5 and #7 (Appendix B-5)

■ Closure of the Session (approximate time: 5 minutes)

a. Summary
b. Homework assignment

Summary: Briefly summarize the major points covered in the body of Session 7 (#2). Ask members if they have any questions.

Homework Assignment: Ask members to continue writing in their journals. Have the women look over past entries and continue to practice the brainstorming and evaluation skills.

★ Remind members of the time and day of the next meeting.

Session Overview

Concept: Confirmation of Choice
- Gather information about actual outcome and consequences of the alternative chosen.
- Make a critical evaluation of the consequences of the choice.
- If goals have been met, exit problem-solving model. If goals have not been met, return to appropriate step of problem-solving model.

Session Objectives
- The client will be able to evaluate the results of their choice by gathering information about actual consequences and outcome.
- The client will be able to evaluate outcomes with regard to formulated goals and expectations.
- Using the information gathered, the client will be able to decide whether the choice was successful or unsuccessful.
- If the choice was unsuccessful, the client will be able to re-enter the appropriate step of the problem-solving model to identify another possible alternative solution to implement.

Session Format
1. Introduction
    a. Review of Session 7
    b. Overview of Session 8
2. Maximizing success
    a. Assess outcomes
    b. Compare outcomes to stated goals
    c. If satisfied, exit the model
    d. If goals have not been met, analyze why
3. Advantages of using the problem-solving model.
    a. Random *versus* planned approaches
    b. Making informed choices
    c. Increased confidence
4. Closure of the session

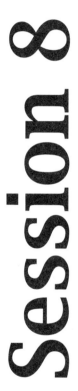

a. Summary

Materials Needed

- Lecture notes
- Blackboard, chalk and eraser, or large sheets of paper, markers, and tacks
- Handout #8 (Appendix B-5)
- Overhead #1 (Appendix C)

■ Introduction (approximate time: 15 minutes)

a. Review of Session 7
b. Overview of Session 8

Summary: Summarize the major points covered in Session 7. You can use Handout #7 (Appendix B-5).

Ask group members if they have any questions or comments. Solicit any input they may have about the homework assignment. How did the journal work for them? Were they able to successfully apply all of the brainstorming rules and evaluate each alternative for their problem situation?

Overview: During today's session, the group will learn about the fifth and final step of the problem-solving model, Confirmation of Choice. This is the final session of the intervention.

■ Maximizing success (approximate time: 30 minutes)

a. Assess outcomes
b. Compare outcomes to stated goals
c. If satisfied, exit the model
d. If goals have not been met, analyze why

Materials Needed

- Lecture notes
- Handout #8 (Appendix B-5)
- Overhead #1 (Appendix C)

Session 8

Lecture Format: Below, a sample lecture is provided for you. Its content covers the major points outlined above. You may use the lecture verbatim or you can use your own words to convey the information. If you choose to use your own words, be careful to cover the major content and themes that are contained in the sample lecture. Midway through the lecture, distribute Handout #8 (Appendix B-5) and display Overhead #1 (Appendix C). The handout contains an outline of the major points. Use this as a visual prompt for the remainder of the lecture.

Sample Lecture: *We are now going to learn about the fifth and final step in the problem-solving model, Confirmation of Choice. This step is used after we have made our choice, developed a plan to put our choice into action, and followed through with whatever action plan we decided on.*

What we do during this last step of the problem-solving model is to evaluate the results that our choice has brought about. This is a very important step that should not be skipped over. Evaluating the outcome of a choice will tell us whether or not our choice was effective, whether or not it worked. If we did not take the time to evaluate, we might continue to make the same kind of choice even when it really had not worked well in solving our problem.

There are three things we must do to find out if our choice was effective. First, we need to gather information about consequences and outcome of our choice. What actually happened as a result of our choice? We should keep a watchful eye on the problem situation. Writing down what we see as consequences of our choice can help us gather information in an organized way. Second, we must evaluate those consequences. Did the outcome match goals and expectations? Are we satisfied with the results of our choice? Has the problem situation improved? If the answer to these questions is "yes," then we have found a good solution to the problem. If the answer to these questions is "no," then our solution is not satisfactory. This would lead us to the third phase of our confirmation process. If our choice has failed to solve the problem, we would want to go back and use the problem-solving model again until a solution that we are happy with is found.

Let's take a look at an outline of Step 5: Confirmation of Choice. We will walk through the guidelines that I have just been talking about using an example.

📄 Distribute Handout #8 (Appendix B-5) and display Overhead #1 (Appendix C) now.

Lesson Plan

Do you remember Sandy? Let me read Sandy's problem to you one more time. We'll give Donna a rest.

Sandy's Problem Situation

Sandy has worked at her job for five years now. It has been a good experience and she has received a lot of positive attention for her efforts. Recently she has felt a little bored and wished she could try something new. When her boss offered her a new and more challenging position in the company, Sandy had mixed feelings. Part of her was excited and happy. Another part of her was afraid. She worried that she did not have the ability to do what her boss was asking. Sandy went home after work consumed and upset by her mixed feelings. Although she had not drank in months, Sandy decided to have a glass of wine to calm her nerves. One drink led to another and before she knew it, Sandy had finished the bottle of wine. The next morning Sandy went to work and turned down the offer of a new position.

Sandy's goal might have been to get a job that was more stimulating and challenging. When offered a position that held the potential to meet her goal, she did not take it because of her mixed feelings. Sandy's solution to her problem was to turn down the position.

Let's look at our handout now. It's difficult to know just what happened with Sandy and how she felt, but let's put our feet in her shoes for a moment and guess how the situation might have turned out for her.

At this point work through each step of the handout with the group, trying to see things from Sandy's point of view. Encourage group participation and give positive reinforcement for sharing ideas. Record their ideas on the blackboard under the appropriate headings.

As demonstrated in the example, we can get a feel for how important it is to evaluate our choices. If Sandy had not taken the time to evaluate her choice, she may have continued to turn down opportunities for a better job.

After evaluating her choice, it is obvious that it did not meet her goal nor was it a choice that brought her satisfaction. When the next opportunity arises she can take a different approach. Like Sandy, we need to take a close look at what our choices bring us. In this way, we always have the opportunity to correct or improve upon those choices that did not work for us. This opens the door to finding a choice that does work.

■ Advantages of Using the Problem-Solving Model (approximate time: 25 minutes)

  a. Random *versus* planned approaches
  b. Making informed choices
  c. Increased confidence

Materials Needed

- Lecture notes
- Blackboard, chalk and eraser, or large sheets of paper, markers, and tacks

Large Group Discussion and Exercise Format: Two exercises, each lasting 10 minutes, will be conducted to cover the content outlined above. The first exercise will be used to help group members contrast random and planned problem-solving approaches and to recognize the advantages in using the problem-solving model they have just learned. Following the first exercise, members will practice seeing themselves as effective and independent problem solvers. A visualization exercise is provided for this purpose. Be sure to slowly read this exercise verbatim, using a calm reassuring tone. Pacing is a very important aspect of relaxation and visualization.

Exercise One: Discussion

Directions: Facilitate the group in comparing and contrasting random and planned problem-solving approaches. Encourage personal comments and insights. Highlight the advantages of using the model they have learned. Record group responses on the blackboard in the format shown below. The displayed format contains some examples of appropriate responses.

Random	Planned
Little initial energy put out.	A moderate amount of energy needed.
A lot of energy put out after the choice is made . . . cleaning up the mess.	Informed choices have a better chance of working.

Exercise Two: Visualization

Directions: *Now I want to invite everybody to do our visualization exercise for the last time. Remember, seeing yourself as an effective problem solver is half of the battle. A little confidence can go a long way. Are you ready? First, I want you to get as comfortable as possible. Take your shoes off if that helps. . . . Good. Now close your eyes, here we go.*

Exercise: *Keeping your eyes closed, I want you to take a few deep breaths . . . slowly breathe in . . . and breathe out . . . inhale . . . exhale. Good. With each breath you feel yourself becoming more and more relaxed . . . more and more calm . . . inhale . . . exhale. That's right. Nothing can disturb your sense of peace . . . and tranquility . . . nothing can bother you . . . there are no pressing matters . . . nothing that needs your attention . . . you are free to relax and enjoy the calm peacefulness . . . with each passing moment . . . you find yourself . . . more and more . . . relaxed. Tension is leaving your body . . . slowly draining away . . . with each breath . . . you feel more and more comfortable . . . more calm. Time loses all meaning for you . . . it no longer matters . . . as you feel the peacefulness gently come over you. You are now entering a different world . . . the road is easy to travel . . . because you feel . . . calm . . . relaxed . . . and successful in the new world. Let your mind take you there . . . your special place where you feel peace and serenity surround you . . . hugging your body . . . your very being. Take a look around you and notice . . . the sights . . . the smells . . . and the sounds. What a wonderful place this is . . . so quiet and peaceful. Enjoy the relaxing atmosphere of your special place . . . in your special place . . . you can deal with anything that happens . . . relaxed . . . confident . . . calm . . . experience the good feelings of success . . . and mastery . . . nothing is impossible . . . you can take care of whatever comes your way . . . when you see a problem coming . . . you are . . . calm and peaceful . . . confident that you can take care of the problem. And you do . . . it feels good to take care of things and move on . . . skilled . . . confident . . . sure of yourself. You did so well . . . you can feel good about your abilities . . . relaxed . . . successful. . . . And now its time to leave your special place . . . you can come back whenever you want . . . you can bring back the good feelings you had . . . in your special place . . . peacefulness . . . strength . . . confidence . . . success. Slowly come back . . . as you become more and more aware of your breathing . . . once again . . . come back. At the count of five. . . . I want you to open your eyes . . . one . . . two . . . three . . . four . . . five . . . now open your eyes.*

Directions: Give the group members a few moments to re-orient themselves. Invite any of the members who would like to comment on their experience to share with the group. How did the exercise work for them this time as compared to the first time they did it?

■ Closure of the Session (approximate time: 15 minutes)

Summary: Briefly summarize the major points covered in the body of Session 8 (#1 through #3). Ask members if they have any questions. Extra time should be allotted during this summary to insure that all questions can be answered and that all concerns can be addressed.

**Appendix A-1 • Session 2
Problem Situation Handout #1**

Janet's boss is a stickler for being on time. Janet knows this and tries to hurry her two elementary schoolers through breakfast so she can get to work on time. The harder she tries, the "behinder" she gets. It is not unusual for Janet to arrive late to work exhausted from her morning battle.

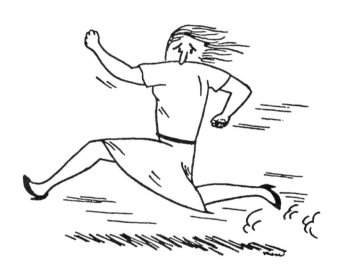

**Appendix A-1 • Session 2
Problem Situation Handout #2**

Janet and Frank would describe their sex life as okay. Since Janet has quit using drugs, she has found herself feeling less and less attracted to her husband. Janet attempts to avoid intimacy with Frank because she is puzzled and confused by these new feelings. Frank has become more aggressive in pursuing a sexual relationship with Janet since she has become distant.

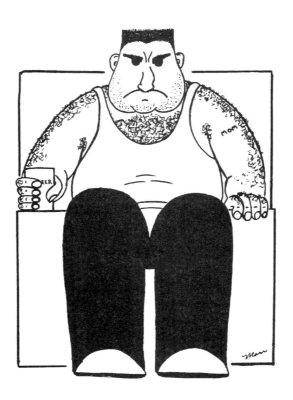

Appendix A   75

Appendix A-2 • Session 2
Role Play #1

Characters: Sue and Janet

Situation: Sue and Janet used to be best friends—used to be, that is until Janet chose to stop drinking. Now the two old friends find themselves in all kinds of conflicts. Today, Sue is very angry because Janet will not agree to go to their old hangout—the corner bar. Sue loses control of her temper, yells at Janet, and accuses her of not caring about their friendship anymore. Sue also accuses Janet of being selfish and snotty.

Questions:

- Who owns the problem?
- What might be behind Sue's anger?

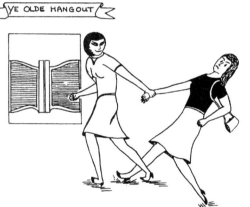

*Instructions: Reproduce each of these statements and cartoons and put on 5 x 8 index cards.

Appendix A-2 • Session 2
Role Play #2

Characters: Janet and Frank

Situation: Janet and Frank have been married for 12 years. Things went O.K. until Janet decided to get a job. Now, when Janet returns home from work, she meets a drunk Frank at the door who demands his dinner immediately. While Janet commutes home from work, Frank sits in front of the television and drinks. Janet wonders aloud why Frank did not fix dinner. With this comment Frank leaves the house in a huff. Janet feels guilty and depressed, wishing she could be a better wife.

Questions:

- Who owns the problem?
- What are the problems?
- What were you thinking and feeling during the role play?

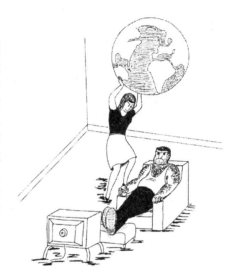

Appendix A-2 • Session 7
Role Play #3

Tina has enjoyed living alone for the past seven years. Recently, finances were such that Tina decided to get a roommate. Things went well for several months as the two roommates got to know each other. But, little by little problems began coming up. Despite Tina's best efforts, things have only gotten worse. Her roommate, Fran, does not always pay her share of the bills on time. Often, Tina ends up paying Fran's share so her credit won't suffer. Fran has also started using drugs in the house despite a promise to Tina that she would not.

Tina now wonders if getting a roommate was such a good idea. She is having a difficult time getting along with Fran. And her money problems are worse than ever.

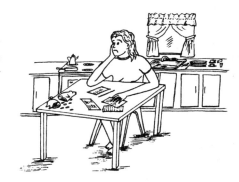

Appendix A-2 • Session 7
Role Play #4

Betty is an outspoken woman who has an opinion about everything. Jill is quiet and a deep thinker. She is not easily swayed by others' opinions but is tolerant of others' views. Betty and Jill have been friends for many years. They grew up together, partied together, and now they are trying to stay sober together.

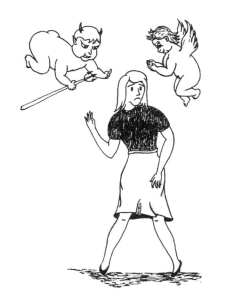

Betty wants Jill to go out to eat with her. The idea sounds great but Jill is down to her last 10 dollars. Payday is three days away. Besides, the restaurant Betty has chosen is more like a bar. There is great temptation for Jill to drink there—the sights, sounds, and smells are all too familiar. Jill tries to politely tell her friend "no thanks," but Betty won't take "no" for an answer. She thinks Jill is being silly . . . scared of her own shadow.

Appendix A-3 • Session 4
Problem Situation #1 Game Card

> Your kids have been driving you crazy lately. It used to be that you could have a few drinks and it didn't matter anymore. But today you have come to realize that drinking did not solve your parenting problems. In fact, your drinking made things worse. Now the kids are difficult to manage and you don't know how to make things better. Your oldest child is often aggressive and angry while the youngest one seems to cry constantly.
>
> You love your kids and want things to get better for them and you. You call the kids' counselor at school hoping she knows of some place that offers parenting classes and family counseling. You remind her of your limited funds!
>
> **Your Goal:** To feel better about your parenting and hopefully see improvement in the behavior of your children.

***Instructions:** Reproduce each of these statements and put on 5 x 8 index cards.

Appendix A-3 • Session 4
Problem Situation #2 Game Card

You and your husband have just celebrated your ninth wedding anniversary. Since marrying him you have stayed home to manage the household, care for the children, and keep the books for the family business. Staying busy is not a problem. Managing stress is. There is always so much to do.

Before you got into treatment and recovery, a few drinks or a tranquilizer relieved your tension and anxiety. Even though your husband disapproved of this practice, there was nobody around to tell him. You always tried to be straight when the children came home from school.

Now, newly recovering, you find that the temptation to use is at its worst during the daytime when you are alone. You know you need help.

Your Goal: To get help during the day.

Appendix A

**Appendix A-3 • Session 4
Problem Situation #1 Sorry Cards**

```
-----------------------------------------
|                                 Problem 1 |
|   Sorry!                                  |
|                                           |
|   Your husband thinks there is nothing wrong |
|   with the kids or your parenting.        |
-----------------------------------------
```

```
-----------------------------------------
|                                 Problem 1 |
|   Sorry!                                  |
|                                           |
|   The kids don't want to talk to some stranger. |
|   They think family counseling is a dumb idea. |
|   After all, you are the one with the problem! |
|   They want you to get a counselor . . . and |
|   leave them out of it.                   |
-----------------------------------------
```

Instructions: Reproduce each of these statements and put on 3 x 5 index cards.

Problem 1

Sorry!

The school counselor says that she does not know where you can get help. She is new in town and does not know of any agencies she can refer you to. Besides, she is swamped.

Problem 1

Sorry!

Your car is not the most reliable in the world. What if it breaks down and you cannot get to the counseling session? Maybe you should wait to get involved in family counseling—at least until you have more reliable transportation.

Problem 1

Sorry!

You are so tired. You want to stay home and rest after a long day. Maybe you can go to parenting classes when you are not so tired.

Appendix A

Problem 1

Sorry!

Family counseling at First Rate Counseling Agency costs $65 per hour . . . way out of your price range.

Problem 1

Sorry!

Your parenting classes are on Wednesday night—the same night your mother plays bridge with her friends. Your mother can't watch the kids for you that night.

Problem 1

Sorry!

Your 12-step sponsor says that your sobriety comes first. She has asked you to attend three meetings per week. Your husband has told you that three nights out is enough—put your parenting concerns on hold.

**Appendix A-3 • Session 4
Problem Situation #2 Sorry Cards**

Problem 2

Sorry!

There are no 12-step meetings during the day in your small town.

Problem 2

Sorry!

Your 12-step sponsor works during the day. She has asked you not to call her during working hours.

Appendix A 85

Problem 2

Sorry!

You need to be home when the kids get home from school. And you must prepare the family meal.

Problem 2

Sorry!

Your parents refuse to believe that you have a problem.

Problem 2

Sorry!

Maybe you are just being silly. Besides, you have work to do and deadlines to meet for the family business.

> **Sorry!**
>
> **Problem 2**
>
> You are without transportation during the day. Your husband takes the family car to work.

> **Sorry!**
>
> **Problem 2**
>
> The neighbor says that she got straight all by herself. If she did not need help, neither do you.

> **Sorry!**
>
> **Problem 2**
>
> Your husband says that you will do fine—you will just have to get used to being alone without drugs. It will just take a little time.

Appendix A

Appendix A-4 • Sessions 4, 6, and 7
Voting Cards

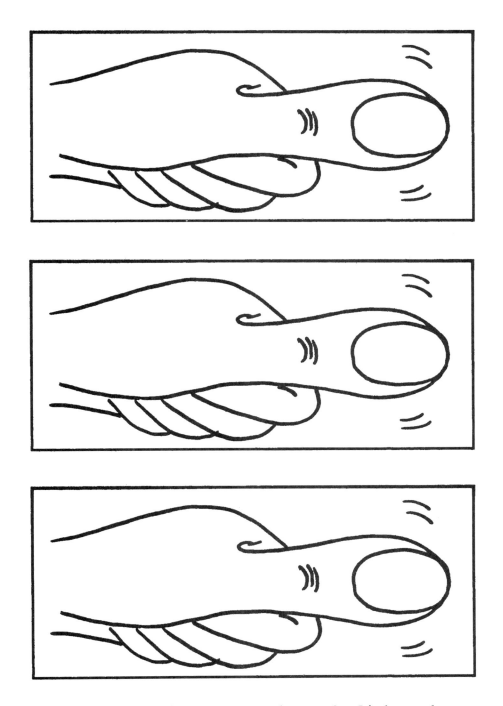

*Instructions: Reproduce each of these cartoons and put on 3 x 5 index cards.

**Appendix B-5 • Session 2
Handout #1**

Problem Situation

Pat is an attractive brunette in her early forties. Since her divorce two years ago, she insists that variety is the all important ingredient in her social life, particularly in dating. Although Pat talks a good line, she is starting to wonder if her version of "variety" is all that great. She has lost count of the number of men she has dated and questions her decision to be intimate with most of them for brief periods of time. When she is honest with herself, she admits that most of the time she feels lonely and abandoned even when she is with one of her men. Pat attempts to erase her feelings of emptiness and fear with more men but the feelings never seem to stay away for long.

Question: What is the main problem?

Question: What are the underlying concerns?

Question: Who owns the problem?

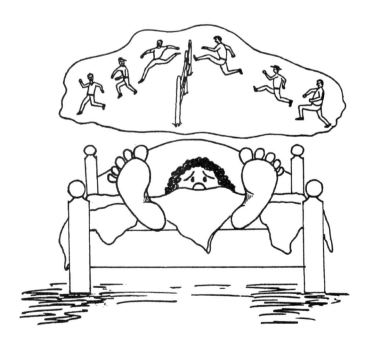

**Appendix B-5 • Sessions 3, 4, and 5
Handout #2**

Version One of Donna's Story

Donna has been staying home a lot lately. Since she quit using, Donna's daily routine includes: taking her two preschoolers to the babysitter's house in the green Ford she drives, going to work at the department store, picking the children up, running errands, returning home to cook for herself and her children, and staying home the remainder of the evening doing household chores. The exception to this routine occurs on Tuesday and Friday nights when Donna attends her 12-step group meetings.

Usually she chooses to go straight home rather than go out for coffee with other members after the meetings. When Donna's old friends or family calls, she keeps conversations short and makes excuses for not visiting with them.

Donna feels tired, lonely, and scared. She worries that she will use again if she does not stay away from her old habits and old friends. Using again could mean that she would lose custody of her two young children. She could not bear this. People in her 12-step group have offered support but Donna's fear has walled her off from their help. Besides, Donna is uncomfortable with the people in her group. Even though attending has helped her to stay drug free, Donna doesn't want to get too involved. She thinks that a lot of the members are very religious and expect her to believe in God.

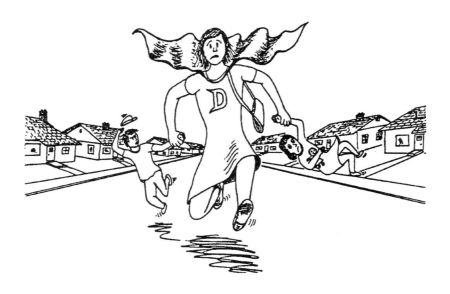

Appendix B-5 • Session 3
Handout #3

Version Two: Donna's Story

Donna doesn't *hang out* much anymore. She just does her *daily stuff*. A *couple* times a week she goes to *meetings*. But that's it.

She's worried about *getting strung out* again and *losing* her kids. Donna just feels *kind of yucky*. She doesn't want help from her group because she's not into that *God stuff*.

Look at Handout #2, "Version One of Donna's Story," to define the terms that are italicized in the story above.

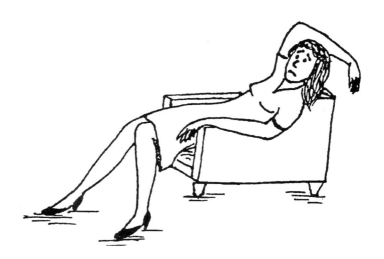

Appendix B-5 • Session 4
Handout #4

Problem Situation
|
Identify

✻ ✻

Concerns	Who Owns It	Stop and Think
• major	?	!
• underlying		

✻ ✻

Define

Important Information	Clearness
• external	• of words used
• internal	• of descriptions
• background	

General Goals	Subproblems
	• obstacles
	• conflicts

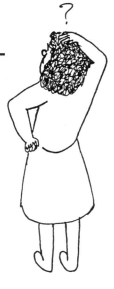

✻ ✻ ✻ ✻ ✻ ✻ ✻ ✻ ✻ ✻ ✻ ✻ ✻ ✻ ✻ ✻ ✻ ✻
✹ ✹ ✹ ✹ **State the Problem** ✹ ✹ ✹ ✹

APPENDIX B-5 • Session 5, 6, and 7
Handout #5

Brainstorming
Brainstorming
Brainstorming Brainstorming
Brainstorming Brainstorming
Brainstorming Brainstorming Brainstorming
Brainstorming Brainstorming Brainstorming
Brainstorming Brainstorming Brainstorming Brainstorming
Brainstorming Brainstorming Brainstorming Brainstorming

The Four Basic Rules of Brainstorming

1. Openness

2. Creativity

3. Quantity

4. Improvement

Brainstorming Brainstorming Brainstorming Brainstorming
Brainstorming Brainstorming Brainstorming Brainstorming
Brainstorming Brainstorming Brainstorming
Brainstorming Brainstorming Brainstorming
Brainstorming Brainstorming
Brainstorming Brainstorming
Brainstorming
Brainstorming

**Appendix B-5 • Session 6
Handout #6**

Alternatives
Evaluation And Decision

1. Select Out Inferior Alternatives

2. Explore Potential Outcomes

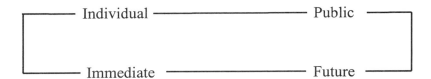

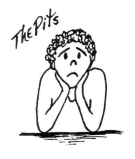

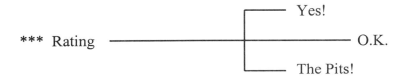

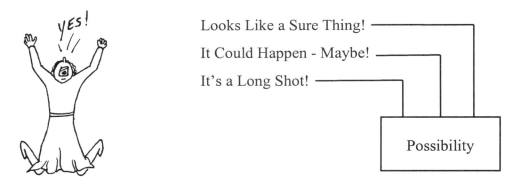

3. Rank the Alternatives (from most to least desirable)

   ❑ Great!
   ❑ Good!
   ❑ O.K.
   ❑ Not So O.K.

4. Make a Decision

Appendix B-5 • Session 7
Handout # 7

Step One: Identify the Problem

Concerns	Who Owns It	Stop and Think
• major • underlying	?	!

Step Two: Define the Problem

Important Information	Clearness
• external • internal • background	• of words used • of descriptions

General Goals	Subproblems
	• obstacles • conflicts

✴ ✴ ✴ ✴ ✴ ✴ ✴ ✴ **State the Problem** ✴ ✴ ✴ ✴ ✴ ✴ ✴ ✴

Step Three: Brainstorm Alternative Solutions
Step Four: Evaluate Alternatives and Make a Decision

Select Out > > > > > > > > > > > > > > > > <u>Explore Potential Outcomes</u>
- Individual • Immediate
- Public • Future

Rating ───┬─ Yes!
             ├─ O.K.
             └─ The Pits!

Looks Like a Sure Thing! ─────┐
It Could Happen – Maybe! ─────┤
It's a Long Shot! ────────────┤
                              │
                         ┌────┴────┐
                         │ Possibility │
                         └─────────┘

Rank the Alternatives (from most to least desirable)

❏ Great!   ❏ O.K.
❏ Good!   ❏ Not so O.K.

Make a Decision

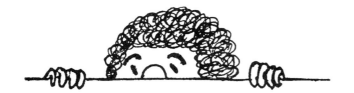

Confirmation of Choice

1. Assess Outcomes

    a. What were the consequences of your choice? What happened?

    b. Write them down.

2. Compare Outcomes to Stated Goals

    a. Did the outcome match well with your goals?

    b. Was the outcome what you predicted?

    c. Are you happy with the outcome?

3. If Satisfied, Exit the Model

    a. If the outcome met your needs and expectations, your problem has been taken care of. See you next time.

4. If Not Satisfied

    a. If the outcome was not to your satisfaction, find out why.

    b. Now, enter the problem-solving model once again to find another solution that may work.

**Appendix C
Sessions 2, 3, and 8
Overhead #1**

Sandy has worked at her job for five years now. It has been a good experience and she has received a lot of positive attention for her efforts. Recently she has felt a little bored and wishes she could try something new. When her boss offers her a new and more challenging position in the company, Sandy has mixed feelings. Part of her is excited and happy. Another part of her is afraid. She is worried that she does not have the ability to do what her boss is asking. Sandy drives home after work consumed and upset by her mixed feelings. Although she has not drank in months, Sandy decides to have a glass of wine to calm her nerves. One drink leads to another and before she knows it, Sandy has finished the bottle of wine. The next morning Sandy returns to work and turns down the offer of a new position.

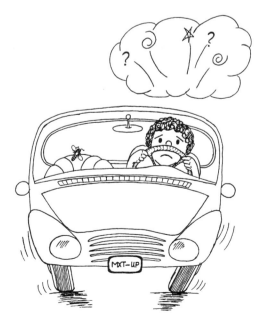

**Appendix C • Session 4
Overhead #2**

You and your husband have just celebrated your ninth anniversary. Since marrying him, you have stayed home to manage the household, care for the children and keep the books for the family business. Staying busy is not a problem. Managing stress is. There is always too much to do.

Before you got into treatment and recovery, a few drinks or a tranquilizer relieved your tension and anxiety. Even though your husband disapproved, nobody was around most of the day to tell him. You always tried to be straight by the time the children came home from school.

Now, newly recovering, you find that temptation to use is at its worst during the daytime when you are alone. You know you need help.

Your Goal: To get help during the day.

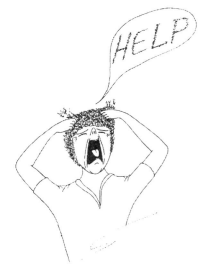

**Appendix C • Session 6
Overhead #3**

Stacey hates to get her mail. It seems like the overdue notices come everyday. She has so many bills that she has lost track of how much she owes and to whom. Her landlord is threatening to evict her and last week the phone service was shut off.

It's not that Stacey doesn't earn a good salary. She does. But Stacey sometimes gets depressed and wants to feel better. A shopping trip usually can pull her right up out of her depression. Shopping works really well until it is over. Then Stacey feels guilty, ashamed, and more depressed than ever. She knows she can't afford her buying sprees. Sometimes Stacey thinks that her money problem is as bad as her drinking problem used to be.

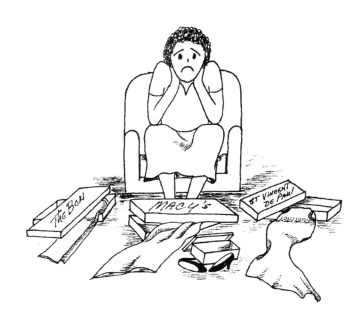

**Appendix D • Session 5
Illustration**

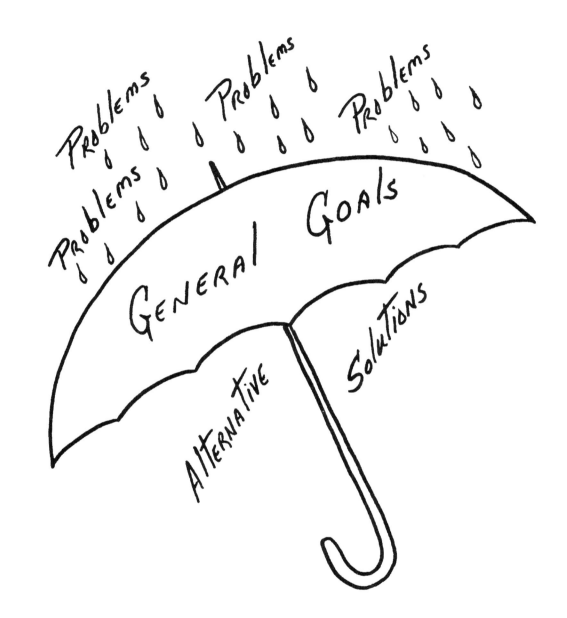

Appendix E
Related Exercises

Gender Specific Treatment is a therapeutic curriculum formatted to teach the basic components of D'Zurilla's and Goldfried's (1971) problem-solving model. It addresses specific skill deficits that pose a barrier to successful resolution of life challenges. Beyond the skills directly related to problem solving are a number of issues that impact the client's ability to transition through each step of the model. Emerging difficulties for a woman in recovery may include a lack of assertiveness, blurred personal boundaries, an inability to trust her inner voice, or an absence of collaboration skills. The following exercises are designed to address issues that may block successful mastery of the skill training concepts.

Issue: Lack of Assertiveness

- **Comments:** When clients lack assertiveness, many potential solutions to the challenges they face seem impossible to implement. It is hard for them to imagine that they possess the personal power to take a stand and follow through effectively. Addressing this issue through awareness training and practice not only equips a woman to make more assertive choices, it increases the probability that she will successfully resolve her presenting problem.

- **Exercise:** Select several issues common to group members and record them on the board. Ask for three volunteers to role play passive, aggressive, and assertive responses. Allow the group to coach the woman who is to make the assertive response. Highlight the differences between passive, aggressive, and assertive responses.

- **Exercise:** After the above role play, send group members home to record situations that arise throughout the week that reflect an opportunity to be assertive. Ask the women to share these with the group. Engage the group in brainstorming different ways to express an assertive response for several of the situations.

- **Exercise:** Get four volunteers up and out of their chairs to create a physical sculpture of passive, aggressive, and assertive responses. One volunteer will act as sculptor while the remaining three will take on an appropriate stance that symbolizes each position. Ask the sculptor to explain why she arranged the volunteers as she did. Solicit responses from the remainder of the group. Finally, invite the "sculpted members" to share their experience. What did they feel in the different positions?

Issue: Blurred Personal Boundaries

- **Comments:** A woman who does not have a clear sense of who she is, or where she ends and another person begins, is likely to have difficulty in accurately identifying who owns a problem. Looking at the continuum of possibilities, personal responsibility may either be exaggerated or totally ignored. The following exercises are designed to assist clients in recognizing and strengthening appropriate personal boundaries.

- **Exercise:** Ask each woman to share an example of a boundary issue they have with a significant other, friend, or co-worker. Highlight the major themes woven across examples. After giving each woman a piece of sidewalk chalk, take the group outside. After discussing possible alternative boundaries, have each woman draw a line on the sidewalk while stating her new boundary aloud. After each woman finishes the exercise, explain how new boundaries can be drawn and improved upon by simply erasing the previous boundary. Flexibility is the essential key as they learn to develop healthier boundaries. Send the women home with the sidewalk chalk, asking them to put it in a place that will help remind them of the importance of boundaries.

- **Exercise:** Use a piece of masking tape to make a line on the floor that represents a personal boundary. Select a group member to stand just behind the line, clearly stating the new boundary she wishes to make. Invite another group member to role play disrespect by crossing the line and clearly stating why they are breaking the boundary. Involve the remainder of the group by having them coach the boundary owner in the following 1) responding in a way that makes it clear that the boundary remains, and 2) describing the consequence for not honoring her boundary.

- **Exercise:** Lead the group in the following cheer. Don't forget to add your own special flair.
  (Spell out) B-O-U-N-D-A-R-I-E-S: Boundaries! Hey!
  Boundaries . . . boundaries . . . they're our friends!
  Serve us well to the end!
  Boundaries . . . boundaries . . . good for us!
  Keeping things healthy is a must!
  Yeaaaaaaaaaaaaaaaaaaaaaaaaaaaah BOUNDARIES!

Issue: Inability to Trust Our Inner Voice

- **Comments:** It is not unusual, particularly for a woman who has been abused, to have difficulty recognizing or trusting her inner voice. Not having a clear sense of who she is in terms of values and beliefs, and lacking positive self-esteem, she ultimately stifles the personal guide that could shape her decisions and actions. Thus she unwittingly allows others to assign values that do not reflect her personal convictions. The following exercises will assist clients in finding and learning to trust their inner voice.

- **Exercise:** Ask the women to list three different occasions when they heard their inner voice but did not heed its directive. In partners, ask group members to explore reasons why they chose to ignore their inner voice. With each pair reporting to the larger group, record themes on one side of the blackboard. On the remaining side, list approaches that can be used to honor our inner voices. For example, by recording its message in a journal and taking a "wait-and-see" attitude, we acknowledge our inner voice without making an ill-planned or hasty choice. With the gift of time, we are likely to discover the intrinsic wisdom that supports a more genuine existence.

- **Exercise:** Ask group members to keep a journal of ways their inner voice speaks to them. Encourage the women to record all incidences they suspect might fall under this category. During the next meeting, ask each woman to share their discoveries and questions with the group. End the exercise by asking members to record on slips of paper, gifts received from their inner voice. Members can then place these in a small attractive gift box that can be taken home as a reminder to honor this part of themselves.

Issue: Deficits in Collaboration

- **Comments:** Given that we typically do not live in isolation, finding solutions to life's challenges often requires collaboration with others. Many women in recovery have come from homes that lacked appropriate models. Either one family member made decisions for the rest of the family, or all members were expected to act as autonomous entities. Learning collaboration skills will assist clients in identifying appropriate solutions that will serve not only themselves, but significant others as well.

- **Exercise:** Using children's puzzles with large pieces, divide each puzzle into two or three piles, placing the pieces in separate envelopes. Ask members to find a partner to work with. Distribute envelopes to each pair with the instructions to do whatever they can to complete their puzzle. After the puzzles have been completed go around the group to discover how members met their goal. Highlight collaborative skills and assist the group in brainstorming other ideas to improve upon their experience.

- **Exercise:** Divide the group into triads to practice basic communication skills. Each group should have one observer, and one "sender" and "receiver" of communication. Basic communication skills that support collaboration include:

    a) listening
    b) physical attending
    c) "I" statements

d) reflection of feelings

e) paraphrase

Define the skill to be practiced and provide an appropriate model. Give the group a problem situation to role play. Each group member should have an opportunity to practice all three of the roles before moving on to the next skill.

Issue: Beliefs that Block Growth

- **Comments:** Many clients cling to irrational beliefs that distort their perspective, creating unnecessary psychological pain, isolation, and misunderstandings. The problems that often result from irrational beliefs can easily be ameliorated by replacing them with more functional beliefs. The following exercise is designed to equip clients to challenge beliefs that no longer serve them well, and replace the beliefs with those that support recovery and facilitate problem solving.

- **Exercise:** Give group members an opportunity to experience irrational beliefs visually. Using samples of various irrational beliefs, sculpt the beliefs by engaging willing group members. Facilitate a group discussion aimed at disputing the irrational belief, then ask a volunteer to sculpt a rational belief using the same willing group members. Allow the group to give input during this process until all members are satisfied with the solution.

Issue: Difficulty with Empathic Understanding

- **Comments:** When successful problem solving requires consideration of several viewpoints, some women in recovery may have difficulty "walking in the shoes" of significant others. The following exercise is designed to shift perception so as to create empathy for those who are affected by a mutually owned problem.

- **Exercise:** Give each woman two masks, one that signifies their public persona, and the other their private selves. Using old magazines, have the group cut out pictures that symbolize parts of these two selves and glue them on to the appropriate mask. After the masks are created, ask each woman to share the meaning of her masks. When all have shared, conduct a group discussion focused on what members learned about each other. Knowing this new information will give them a greater understanding of how others experience the world.

- **Exercise:** Ask group members to remove their shoes, place them in a pile on the floor, then sit in a circle around the pile. Going around the circle, ask each woman select a shoe, inspect it, and imagine what the shoe has experienced by traveling with another woman. Finally, ask the women to tell a short story about the life of their shoe. At the end of the exercise, emphasize the idea that everyone has a unique story to tell, a life history that can only be discovered as we train our attention on the other person. Understanding others requires energy and effort on our part.

Issue: Managing Conflict

- **Comments:** Many women try to avoid conflict for a variety reasons. Difficulty in managing conflicts can severely impair the problem-solving process. If mutual solutions are to be identified, women in recovery will need the skills to first appropriately disagree, and then forge a compromise with others. The following exercises are designed to increase comfort with conflict, and develop skills that lead to resolution.

- **Exercise:** Working in partners, ask each woman to briefly describe a conflict they have experienced. Using a large sheet of paper, diagram each conflict using the following categories:

  a) presenting conflict;
  b) group member's view of the issue;
  c) opposing party's view of the issue;
  d) each party's extenuating circumstances that, in some way, impact the conflict;
  e) each party's desired solution;
  f) possible common ground;
  g) area of possible compromise.

  After diagraming the conflict, ask the partners to develop a list of plausible solutions.

- **Exercise:** Discuss the impact of negative nonverbal language and inflammatory vocabulary on problem situations.* Ask the group to select several typical conflicts that might occur in recovery. Using the examples, have members role play a conflict-inspiring response and a conflict-soothing response. Highlight the contrast between each stance.

Issue: Voices from the Past

- **Comments:** It is not unusual for "old tapes" to color the vision a woman has for her present as well as her future. Voices from the past often carry judgmental and inaccurate statements about who she is, what she can become, and what she should and should not do. Learning to recognize these voices and challenge their edicts will assist every woman in recovery to make new choices, and thus craft a new vision for her life. The following exercises are designed to

---

*Inflammatory language is not limited to vulgar expressions. Vocabulary used in normal situations may be viewed as inflammatory. How we express a thought can make all the difference in the world. Consider the following example: a) Your child is stingy and spoiled, b) Your child sometimes has difficulty sharing the toys.

facilitate recognition of "old tapes," the power they have held, and the possibility of their elimination.

- Exercise: Ask group members to record individual messages from the past on separate pieces of paper, then sort into the following categories: 1) who she is, 2) what she can become, and 3) what she should and should not do. Position a large waste can in the middle of the group and then ask women to come up one at a time to read the messages. After they read the message, ask them to crumble up the paper, throw it in the trash can, and boldly repeat the following statements for each corresponding category.

- **Statements:** 1) Not! I have the power to choose who I am today; 2) Not! I can discover my gifts and talents, using them to pursue my interests and dreams; 3) Not! I have the power to decide what is right for me today.

  Encourage the group to verbally support each other during the exercise. After the last member has completed the exercise, allow the group to discuss the experience. What impact has the exercise had on feelings and beliefs?

- **Exercise:** Ask the group to craft a bold assertive statement about "old tapes" and the people who sent them inappropriate or damaging messages. Record the statement on the blackboard for all to see. Give each group member an old video or audio cassette. As they enthusiastically repeat their proclamation, have them destroy their tape by pulling it out of its casing. Following this exercise, ask each member to share two "old tapes" they are prepared to discard in the coming week.

Issue: Nurturing Resiliency

- **Comments:** Many women in recovery have no clear sense of the character strengths they possess and often feel helpless when addressing the challenges that confront them. The exercises below are designed to both assist in the identification of personal assets and resources, and teach clients how to build a resilient foundation from which they can address problems.

- **Exercise:** Using a long piece of butcher paper placed on the floor and several different types of creative media (crayons, chalk, pastels, markers, glitter, glue, pipe cleaners, cotton balls), engage the women in creating a group mural with the following theme: children at play. Direct members to draw themselves as the children they know they could have been had they grown up in a perfect and functional world. Play soft background music (without lyrics) throughout the exercise. The exercise is complete when the group agrees that they are finished with the mural. Typically, you will observe a slowing of activity after approximately 30 to 45 minutes. Use the following structure to guide the activity:
a) Group members are to refrain from talking to each other.
b) The use of written language is also prohibited.

c) Group members are encouraged to add features to other member's drawings. This can be done by using nonverbal language to gain permission.
d) Group members are encouraged to allow the playful child within to express herself.

When group members have completed the mural, ask each woman to describe the following:

a) Her general experience in creating the mural.
b) The activities depicted by her drawings.
c) The resiliency characteristics of the child she drew.

Facilitate a discussion about developing the resiliency characteristics of "the child within."

- **Exercise:** Provide a list of resiliency characteristics from which members can choose two traits they wish to develop. With a partner, ask the women to create an action plan to achieve their goals. When the members are finished, ask them to share their ideas with the group. Encourage them to incorporate the ideas they found most attractive into their own action plan.

Issue: Managing Ego Defense Mechanisms

- **Comments:** Ego defense mechanisms are helpful in that they prevent us from being overwhelmed by threatening material. However, they can become problematic if overused. The following exercises help clients to identify the different defense mechanisms they may rely on, and equip them to determine when defenses are overused in an unhealthy way.

- **Exercise:** Give clients a list of defense mechanisms that includes a description and an example of each. Divide the group into teams of four, assigning several defense mechanisms to each team. Ask the teams to create role plays that depict how each defense mechanism might manifest itself in the lives of recovering women. After each role play, ask the remainder of the group to identify the defense mechanism. Allow time for comments and discussion. In particular, give some examples that depict the overuse of each mechanism, highlighting behaviors that can be a cause for concern.

- **Exercise:** Give group members a picture of a gauge. Have the women fasten a moveable paper pointer at the center of the gauge, and draw in areas that signify various degrees of overuse, normal use, and under use. Reviewing the names and meanings of each defense mechanism, ask the women to judge their level of use for each when coping with life challenges. Invite the group to make comments, provide examples, or ask questions about each defense mechanism.

Appendix F
References

Bedell, J. R., R. P. Archer, and H. A. Marlowe. "A Description and Evaluation of a Problem-Solving Skills Training Program." In D. Upper and S. M. Moss (eds.), *Behavioral Group Therapy* (1980): 3-35.

Chaney, E. F., M. R. O'Leary, and G. A. Marlatt. "Skill Training with Alcoholics." *Journal of Counseling and Clinical Psychology* 46/5 (1978): 1092-1104.

Connors, G. J., and K. S. Wallitzer. "Reducing Alcohol Consumption Among Heavily Drinking Women: Evaluating the Contributions of Life-Skills Training and Booster Sessions." *Journal of Consulting and Clinical Psychology* 69/3 (2001): 447-56.

D'Zurilla, T. J., and M. R. Goldfried. "Problem Solving and Behavior Modification." *Journal of Abnormal Psychology* 78 (1971): 107-26.

D'Zurilla, T. J., and A. Nezu. "A Study of the Generation-of-Alternatives Process in Social Problem Solving." *Cognitive Therapy and Research* 4 (1980): 67-72.

Edelstein, B. A., E. Couture, M. Cray, P. Dickens, and N. Lusenbrink. "Group Training of Problem Solving with Psychiatric Patients." In D. Upper and S. M. Ross (eds.), *Behavioral Group Therapy* (1980): 85-101.

Heppner, P. P. "A Review of the Problem-Solving Literature and Its Relationship to the Counseling Process." *Journal of Counseling Psychology* 25 (1978): 366-75.

Hermalin, J., S. Husband, and J. J. Platt. "Reducing the Costs of Employee Alcohol and Drug Abuse: Problem-Solving and Social Skills Training for Relapse Prevention." *Employee Assistance Quarterly* 6/2 (1990): 11-25.

Intagliata, J. C. "Increasing the Interpersonal Problem-Solving Skills of an Alcoholic Population." *Journal of Consulting and Clinical Psychology* 46 (1978): 489-98.

Kelly, M. L., W. O. Scott, D. M. Prue, and R. Rychtarik. "A Component Analysis of Problem-Solving Skills Training." *Cognitive Therapy and Research* 9/4 (1985): 429-41.

Maisto, S. A., G. J. Connors, and W. H. Zywiak. "Alcohol Treatment Changes in Coping Skills, Self-Efficacy, and Levels of Alcohol Use and Related Problems One Year Following

Treatment Initiation." *American Psychological Association/Educational Publishing Foundation* 14/3 (2000): 257-66.

Marr, D. D. "The Effect of a Problem-Solving Strategy Intervention on the Self-Esteem of Chemically Dependent Women in Recovery." *Dissertation Abstracts International,* 52 7A (University Microfilms No. 91-35959), 1991.

Marr, D. D., and T. N. Fairchild. "A Problem-Solving Strategy and Self-Esteem in Recovering Chemically Dependent Women." *Alcoholism Treatment Quarterly* 10/1-2 (1993): 171-86.

Marr, D. D. "Gender Specific Treatment for Chemically Dependent Women: A Rationale for Inclusion of Vocational Services." *Alcoholism Treatment Quarterly* 14/1 (1996): 21-31.

Osborn, A. F. *Applied Imagination: Principles and Procedures of Creative Problem Solving,* 3rd ed. New York: McGraw-Hill, 1963.

Platt, J. J., W. C. Scura, and J. R. Hannon. "Problem-Solving Thinking of Youthful Incarcerated Heroin Addicts." *Journal of Community Psychology* 1 (1973): 273-81.

Straussner, Shulamith Lala Ashenbert (ed.). *The Handbook of Addiction Treatment for Women.* San Francisco: Josey-Bass/Pffeifer, 2002.